ORTHOSTATIC HYPOTENSION

ORTHOSTATIC HYPOTENSION

IRWIN J. SCHATZ, M.D.
Professor and Chairman
Department of Medicine
John A. Burns School of Medicine
University of Hawaii
Honolulu, Hawaii

F. A. Davis Company/PHILADELPHIA

Printed in the United States of America

NOTE: As new scientific information becomes available through basic and clinical research, recommended treatments and drug therapies undergo changes. The author and publisher have done everything possible to make this book accurate, up-to-date, and in accord with accepted standards at the time of publication. However, the reader is advised always to check product information (package inserts) for changes and new information regarding dose and contraindications before administering any drug. Caution is especially urged when using new or infrequently ordered drugs.

Library of Congress Cataloging-in-Publication Data

Schatz, Irwin J., 1931-
Orthostatic hypotension.

Includes bibliographies and index.
1. Hypotension, Orthostatic. I. Title. [DNLM: 1. Hypotension, Orthostatic. WG 340 S312o]
RC685.H93S33 1986 616.1'3 85-29184
ISBN 0-8036-7737-5

To Barbara, Jacob, Edward,
Stephen, and Brian

PREFACE

Dizziness and fainting are ubiquitous symptoms. Physicians faced with helping patients with such complaints must sift through a lengthy list of potential causes. The initial history often provides the physician enough clues so that the course and treatment are obvious. There remains, nevertheless, a group of patients in whom the reason for fainting or dizziness is obscure. In some, even though there may be evidence of a drop in blood pressure on standing, subsequent diagnostic and management paths are uncertain.

Although orthostatic hypotension—low blood pressure when upright—is an important cause of symptoms of cerebral hypoxia, its prevalence in the general population is unknown. Data from the United States are incomplete. For example, evaluation of a group of patients who presented to the emergency room or for hospital admission because of syncope revealed orthostatic hypotension as a cause in 7 percent (14 of 204 cases).[1] Clearly, such a series is self-selected for severity and excludes persons with orthostatic hypotension who might not have fainted but still had cerebral hypoxia, or instead had sought advice in a physician's office.

Similarly, evidence from Europe is anecdotal and indicates that the *diagnosis* of orthostatic hypotension is made frequently. Ray[2] suggests that in Germany the diagnosis is made in 10 to 17 percent of all patient contacts!

Orthostatic hypotension may be caused by a wide spectrum of conditions—ranging from simple, prolonged bed rest to progressive, degenerative central nervous system disease. The physician may be dealing, therefore, with an innocuous and self-limiting physiologic aberration at the one extreme or a debilitating and remorseless affliction at the other.

How does one approach such patients? What diagnostic maneuvers are reasonable to distinguish these various causes? What is the natural history of these disorders? And finally, what advice do we give to our patients? In some cases, simple physical measures are enough to alleviate the symptoms. If they are not, however, how do we decide among the various forms of pharmacologic therapies that have been recommended, and when should they be instituted? The results of some studies imply that certain types of autonomic derangements respond better to specific forms of medical therapy than others. Since the implications for such conclusions are important, what data are available to support them?

This monograph attempts to provide answers to these questions. A description of the normal physiology of blood pressure maintenance upon standing is followed by a discussion of the pathophysiology of both the functional and organic disturbances of these homeostatic mechanisms. Analysis of those syndromes that lead to postural hypotension is provided, followed by a detailed discussion of current concepts in the management of these disorders.

As a result of the interdisciplinary nature of the symptoms of orthostatic hypotension, general internists as well as family practitioners often manage these patients. In addition, the range of presenting symptoms mandates that such patients are frequently referred to specialists, particularly neurologists, cardiologists, urologists, and otolaryngologists. The aim of this monograph is to provide all these concerned clinicians with a central source of information about orthostatic hypotension.

I.J.S.

REFERENCES

1. Kapoor, WN, Karpf, M, Wieand, S, Peterson, JR, Levey, GS: *A prospective evaluation and follow-up of patients with syncope.* N Engl J Med 309:197–204, 1983.

2. Ray, KA: *Symptomatic orthostatic essential hypotension.* Br J Clin Pr 1:265–268, 1983.

ACKNOWLEDGMENTS

This monograph would not have been completed without the early encouragement of Dean Terence A. Rogers, the administrative aid of Naomi Leong, and, in particular, the invaluable secretarial assistance of Sharon Chun.

Susie Anderson contributed medical illustrations of the highest caliber, and Linda Weinerman and Sylvia Fields of the F. A. Davis Company were always helpful and supportive.

Finally, my family exhibited patience and understanding for which I am most grateful.

I.J.S.

CONTENTS

CHAPTER 1. THE MAINTENANCE OF NORMAL BLOOD PRESSURE UPON STANDING 1

Reflex Arteriolar Constriction 2
Reflex Venous Constriction 6
Increase in Heart Rate 6
Hormonal Responses 8
Cerebral Blood Flow 9
Respiratory and Muscle Changes 10

CHAPTER 2. ORTHOSTATIC HYPOTENSION DUE TO FUNCTIONAL DERANGEMENTS 13

Inadequate Postural Adjustment 15
- Asthenic Habitus With Poorly Developed Musculature 15
- Physical Exertion 15
- Bed Rest and/or Space Flight 15
- Aging 16
- Miscellaneous Causes 17

Reduced Effective Circulatory Blood Volume 18
Pharmacologic Agents 19
Miscellaneous Causes 20

CHAPTER 3. ORTHOSTATIC HYPOTENSION DUE TO ORGANIC DERANGEMENTS 25

Neurogenic Orthostatic Hypotension 26

Afferent Lesions 27
Central Disorders 29
Idiopathic Parkinsonism 29
Riley-Day Syndrome (Familial Dysautonomia) 30
Miscellaneous Causes 30
Efferent Defects 31
Idiopathic Orthostatic Hypotension 34
Multiple-System Atrophy (Shy-Drager Syndrome) 35
Clinical Description 35
Natural History 37
Pathology and Pathogenesis of Multiple-System Atrophy and Idiopathic Orthostatic Hypotension 38
Orthostatic Hypotension Associated With Excessive Sympathetic Discharge (Sympathicotonic Orthostatic Hypotension) 41
Orthostatic Hypotension and Mitral Valve Prolapse 42
Miscellaneous Lesions in the Spinal Cord 44
Disorders Primarily Affecting Sympathetic Chain and Postganglionic Nerves 44
Diabetes Mellitus 44
Miscellaneous Neuropathies 45
Defects in Peripheral Vasculature 47
Hyperbradykininism 47
Congenital Defect in Norepinephrine Release 48

CHAPTER 4. NEUROGENIC ORTHOSTATIC HYPOTENSION: PATHOPHYSIOLOGIC AND PHARMACOLOGIC INVESTIGATIONS 55

Studies of Plasma Catecholamines 57
Infusion of Pressor Agents 59

Postsynaptic Adrenergic Receptors 61
Antidiuretic Hormone (Arginine Vasopressin) 61
Enzyme Measurements 62
Studies of Other Pressor Agents 62

CHAPTER 5. CLINICAL DIAGNOSIS 67
Symptoms of Inadequate Arterial Perfusion 69
Symptoms of Autonomic Dysfunction 70
Clinical Diagnosis in the Patient With Orthostatic Hypotension 72
Physical Examination 74
Laboratory Investigations 76
Tests of Autonomic Function 78
- Valsalva Maneuver 78
- Modified Noninvasive Valsalva Maneuver 81

Tests of Afferent Function 81
- Heart Rate Response to Standing 81
- Amyl Nitrate Inhalation 82
- Phenylephrine Hydrochloride Injection 83
- Vasopressin Response to Standing 83

Tests of Central Function 83
Tests of Efferent Function 84
- Noninvasive Tests 84
  - Cold Pressor Test 84
  - Arithmetic Under Stress 84
  - Sweat Tests 84
  - Epinephrine Instillation into the Eye 85
  - Plasma Norepinephrine Levels 85
- Invasive Tests 86
  - Tyramine Infusion 86
  - Norepinephrine Infusion 86

The Clinical Use of Autonomic Function Testing 87

CHAPTER 6. **MANAGEMENT 91**

General Measures 93
Physical Measures 95
Head-Up Tilt at Night 95
Lower Body External Pressure 95
Pharmacologic Measures 97
Fludrocortisone Acetate 98
Vasopressors 100
Ergot Derivatives 102
Prostaglandin Inhibition 105
Adrenergic Blockers 105
Miscellaneous Agents 107
Mechanical Devices 108

CHAPTER 7. **ILLUSTRATIVE CASES 113**

Case 1: Orthostatic Hypotension Induced by Drugs in an Elderly Patient 114
Case 2: Mitral Valve Prolapse, and Sympathicotonic Orthostatic Hypotension 115
Case 3: Diabetic Neuropathy 116
Case 4: Multiple-System Atrophy (Shy-Drager Syndrome) 117
Case 5: Idiopathic Orthostatic Hypotension 119
Case 6: Amyloid Neuropathy 120
Case 7: Carotid Sinus Obliteration 121
Case 8: Multiple-System Atrophy (Shy-Drager Syndrome) 122

EPILOGUE 125

INDEX 127

CHAPTER 1

THE MAINTENANCE OF NORMAL BLOOD PRESSURE UPON STANDING

REFLEX ARTERIOLAR CONSTRICTION

REFLEX VENOUS CONSTRICTION

INCREASE IN HEART RATE

HORMONAL RESPONSES

CEREBRAL BLOOD FLOW

RESPIRATORY AND MUSCLE CHANGES

An exquisite series of physiologic adjustments, designed to maintain cerebral blood flow, occurred when primates first assumed the upright position. Otherwise, there would have been excessive pooling of blood in the peripheral veins, with a consequent substantial reduction in central blood volume, left ventricular filling pressure, cardiac output, and cerebral perfusion. Gauer[1] estimates that there is an immediate loss of approximately 400 ml of blood from the intrathoracic compartment upon standing. Additionally, the initial increase of hydrostatic pressure causes a sudden influx of blood filling the venous system; within 1 to 2 minutes, the venous valves are stretched open and the venous pressure in the feet rises up to 100 mm Hg.[2] This

TABLE 1-1. Physiologic Responses That Maintain Blood Pressure Upon Standing

Reflex arteriolar constriction
Reflex venous constriction (probable)
Reflex acceleration of heart rate
Increase in plasma catecholamines
Activation of renin–angiotensin–aldosterone system
Release of arginine vasopressin
Decrease in cerebral vascular resistance
Augmentation of respiration
Increased striated muscle tone

change in pressure may cause a volume increase of approximately 200 cm^3.

These effects of gravity stimulate a prompt and complex mix of central nervous system (CNS), hemodynamic, and hormonal responses (Table 1-1).

Standing evokes different cardiovascular compensatory mechanisms, depending upon whether there is active or passive muscle use. Borst and coworkers[3] demonstrated that 70-degree head-up tilt ("passive standing") causes a slow, gradual increase in heart rate and blood pressure (BP), whereas immediate ("active") standing results in a modest decrease in BP within 3 to 7 seconds, and a large bimodal increase in heart rate within 3 to 30 seconds. Both of these effects are presumably associated with skeletal muscle contraction (Fig. 1-1). "Active" standing obviously closely simulates normal human activity.

Wieling, Dambrink, and Borst[4] have speculated that the immediate drop in BP is caused by reflex vasodilatation, but loss of central blood volume with a consequent less effective preload is an equally tenable explanation. In any case, the baroreflex response plays a paramount role in subsequent homeostasis.

REFLEX ARTERIOLAR CONSTRICTION

Reflex arteriolar constriction may be the single most important mechanism that operates to maintain BP on stand-

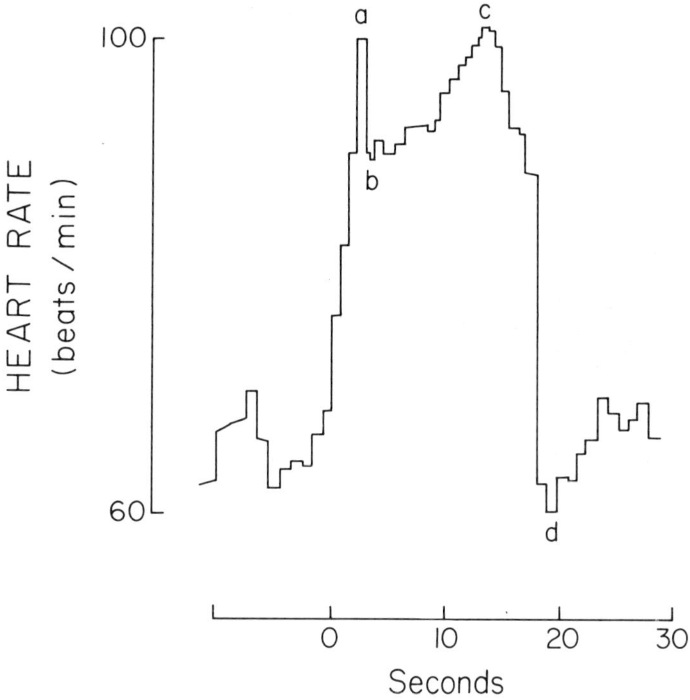

FIGURE 1-1. Example of heart rate response to standing after 30 seconds. Initial response is bimodal; *a* and *c* denote primary and secondary peaks, *b* and *d* indicate primary and secondary valleys, respectively. (Modified and reprinted from Borst, et al,[3] with permission.)

ing. It is mediated through the arterial baroreceptor reflex. When pressure-sensing areas in the intima of the aortic arch, carotid sinus, and the cardiac chambers are stimulated by an increase in BP, there is a subsequent inhibition of sympathetic discharge from these areas (Fig. 1-2). Obviously, therefore, when the opposite occurs—any decrease in stimulation of the arterial baroreceptors, derived from a drop in BP—there results an increase in sympathetic activity, leading to peripheral arterial constriction. This happens principally in the limbs,[5] the splanchnic vasculature,[6] the kidneys,[7] and the lungs.[8]

The reflex arc consists of a somatic afferent pathway, several integrating centers in the brain and spinal cord, and sympathetic as well as parasympathetic outflow through two

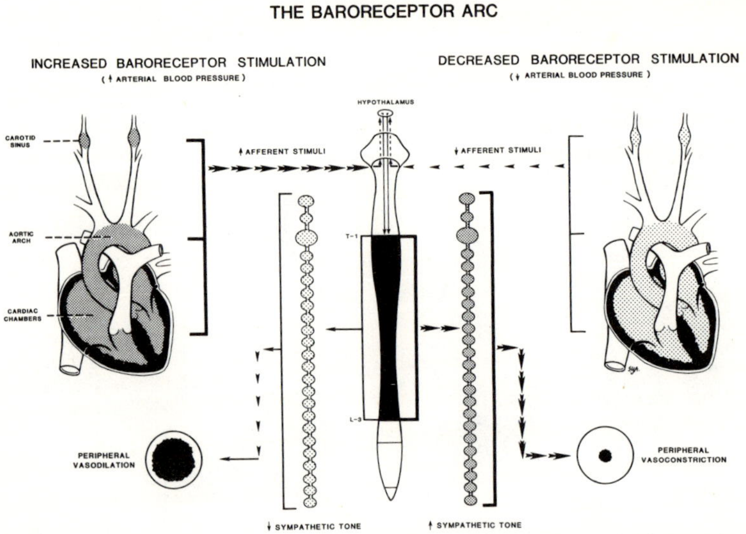

FIGURE 1-2. Schematic representation of the baroreceptor reflex arc.

distinct systems. The afferent pathways course through cranial nerves IX and X and the carotid sinus nerve to enter the CNS and terminate in the brain stem (tractus solitarius and the paramedian nucleus of the reticular formation). These critically important neuronal areas make connections with higher structures in the brain, including the hypothalamus, cerebellum, substantia nigra, and cerebral hemispheres.[9] Complex connections modify and integrate segmental reflexes, and probably involve both excitatory and inhibitory pathways.

Efferent outflow from the midbrain is likely multisynaptic, finally reaching the intermediolateral nucleus of the spinal cord, coursing through the intermediolateral gray column of the spinal cord. The efferent sympathetic pathway leaves the cord through the thoracolumbar outflow (twelfth thoracic and first and second lumbar) as preganglionic myelinated fibers and forms synaptic junctions in prevertebral and trunk ganglia. Postganglionic unmyelinated fibers then join the voluntary motor fibers distributed through these nerves to the blood vessels and organs in the periphery.[9]

It is clear that there is a system of noradrenergic neurons that participate in BP control; these are located both in the periphery[10] and in the brain stem and spinal cord. The preganglionic neurons are cholinergic, whereas the postganglionic nerves are noradrenergic.[9] Bannister points out, however, that the distinction between peripheral sympathetic and parasympathetic systems is difficult to make, since not all the cells in the sympathetic ganglia are adrenergic, and cholinergic muscle vasodilator neurons exist.[11] Additionally, norepinephrine may act not only directly as a transmitter but indirectly by modulating the effect of acetylcholine.[11] There are conflicting data about the precise mechanisms by which these neurons influence autonomic function.[9]

The postsynaptic neurons terminate in a sympathetic varicosity that exists in conjunction with the vascular smooth muscle membrane (Fig. 1-3). These neurons liberate norepinephrine as a neural transmitter; this, then, causes alpha-adrenergic effects (mediated principally through alpha receptors located on the postsynaptic cleft), and beta-adrenergic effects (through beta receptors). The alpha-adrenergic stimulation causes vasoconstriction. Beta stimulation results in not only some vasodilatation in muscles but also an increase in inotropic and chronotropic cardiac activity.

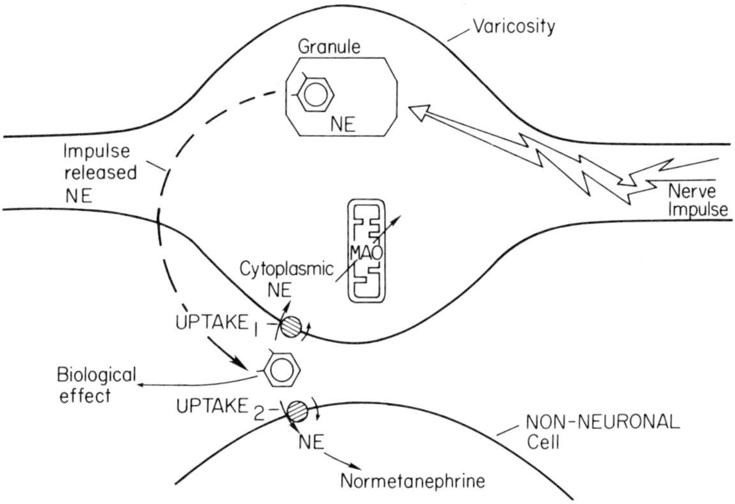

FIGURE 1-3. Schematic representation of the postsynaptic sympathetic varicosity (see text for details).

The efferent parasympathetic pathway leaves the CNS through both cranial and sacral outflow. Preganglionic parasympathetic fibers extend to the ganglia located near or within the organs supplied; postganglionic fibers are short and liberate acetylcholine at the terminal synapse; vagal outflow innervates cardiac, pulmonary, and upper abdominal organs. Pelvic organs are supplied by the sacral outflow.

REFLEX VENOUS CONSTRICTION

As discussed above, massive pooling of blood in the lower extremities results in a marked decrease in central blood volume. This would occur if the veins were merely passive receptacles. Although Bevegard[12] states that there is little evidence that changes in venous tone play a major role, there are abundant data that reflex venous constriction does occur, simultaneous with the increase in peripheral resistance provided by changes in arterial tone.[13]

In a series of elegant studies, Page and colleagues[13] clearly demonstrated that the veins constrict, in response to a number of physiologic influences, including the Valsalva maneuver, tilting, cold, exercise, and hyperventilation. They also showed that in patients considered to have postural hypotension, there was little or no in vitro or in vivo venomotor activity as a response to these stimuli.[13] In normal individuals, peripheral venous constriction causes blood to be shifted to more distensible central portions of the venous system, resulting in an increase in left ventricular filling pressure.

INCREASE IN HEART RATE

The initial heart rate response to standing is derived from a complex series of events involving muscle sensors, high-pressure and low-pressure receptors, and plasma catecholamines.

Recent investigations by Borst and coworkers[3] indicate that this response varies in intensity, duration, and mechanism depending upon whether the standing is active or passive. With active standing, there is an immediate bimodal tachycardia lasting 20 seconds. The response during the first 5 seconds is probably caused by contraction of skeletal muscle groups ("the exercise reflex") and consequent vagal inhibition.[14] This is followed by a secondary cardiac acceleration between 5 and 12 seconds after standing. Because of the close temporal relation between the fall in BP and this secondary tachycardia, the baroreceptor reflex is probably responsible, principally mediated through vagal suppression of sinus node activity.[3,15]

Head-up tilt ("passive" standing) causes a gradual increase of heart rate, unlike that described above (Fig. 1-4). This is likely due to both enhanced sympathetic and decreased parasympathetic cardiac stimulation.[16] Conclusions about the *physiology* of BP control based upon tilt-table studies may be misleading; normal people do not use a tilt-table to stand up, and it is clear from Borst's studies that BP

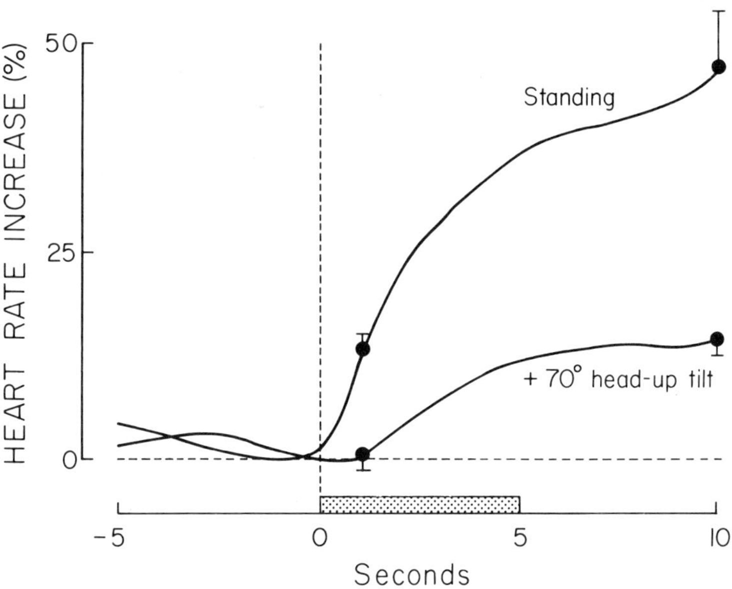

FIGURE 1-4. More gradual increase in heart rate induced by head-up tilt compared with that caused by standing. (Modified and reprinted from Borst, et al,[3] with permission.)

homeostasis when one stands is different from what happens when one becomes passively upright on a tilt-table.

HORMONAL RESPONSES

On standing, an immediate twofold to fourfold increase in plasma norepinephrine occurs, the principal source of which is very likely the sympathetic ganglia, and is a reflection of enhanced sympathetic activity. The adrenal medulla may also participate slightly. As described above, stimulation of the sympathetic terminal varicosity results in norepinephrine release from the granular pool. Some of this is recaptured by the neuron, but significant quantities are O-methylated to form normetanephrine, which is excreted in the urine as VMA (vanillylmandelic acid, or 3-methoxy-4-hydroxymandelic acid).[17] Thus, the measurement of urinary VMA reflects activation of norepinephrine. Additionally, the enzyme dopamine beta-hydroxylase, which converts dopamine to norepinephrine, is also secreted. It has been suggested that other peptides, such as the endogenous opioids, also play a role in BP control; this theory is based on data from animal experiments.[20–22]

The renin–angiotensin–aldosterone system becomes activated and causes renal retention of sodium and water and therefore an increase in blood volume. It is doubtful, however, that this mechanism plays an important role in the immediate adjustment of BP; Guyton[19] has suggested that this more likely is a long-term control mechanism.

Share has pointed out that arginine vasopressin is released from the neurohypophysis in response to rather small changes in blood volume.[23] This feedback loop is achieved by changes in the activity of atrial stretch receptors and arterial baroreceptors (volume receptors). The precise action of this powerful substance in the regulation of cardiovascular hemodynamics and in the maintenance of BP has not been clearly outlined; accumulated data indicate, however, that these so-called volume receptors may play an important role, particularly in controlling long-term responses to changes in intravascular volume.

CEREBRAL BLOOD FLOW

There is a striking capability in normal subjects for autoregulation of the cerebral circulation. As systemic BP falls, cerebral blood vessels dilate so that blood flow is not reduced significantly until mean arterial pressure falls to below 60 mm Hg.[24,25] Below this level, blood flow declines rapidly.

The teleologic explanation for this remarkable capability in maintaining cerebral arterial perfusion must rest with the fact that the brain has no store of high-energy phosphate compounds. Decreased cerebral oxygenation quickly leads to depletion of these substances and consequent cellular dysfunction and unconsciousness.[26] Fortunately, consciousness returns rapidly when adequate oxygen delivery is restored.

Cerebral blood flow is determined by the perfusion pressure (arterial minus venous pressure) and vascular resistance. Since venous pressure in the human cerebral circulation is very low (± 5 mm Hg), arterial pressure essentially determines perfusion pressure.[27]

In normal recumbent subjects, hypoxia becomes manifest at a mean arterial pressure of 40 mm Hg, whereas 60 mm Hg is necessary in the upright position. Because the base of the brain is about 24 cm above the heart, the mean arterial pressure that effectively perfuses the brain is approximately 20 mm Hg less than the actual mean arterial pressure. Measurements of cerebral blood flow in the recumbent and standing positions indicate that there is a decrease of about 20 percent when a subject becomes upright.[28]

Because cerebral blood flow may not change appreciably even though there are remarkable changes in cerebral perfusion pressure (mean arterial pressure), it is likely that cerebrovascular resistance is the most significant determinant of cerebral blood flow. This is almost certainly true when mean arterial pressure is maintained above 60 mm Hg. Although there are many determinants of cerebral vascular resistance (the physical properties of the blood vessels, blood viscosity, and temperature), the most important are the levels of carbon dioxide (P_{CO_2}) and the blood pH. Thus, cerebral blood flow is probably mediated by exquisite sensitivity to changes in levels of these two parameters. In addition, there is some evidence that sympathetic pathways to cerebral vessels from the brain must be intact in order for autoregulation to function properly, but the dimensions of this contribution to control of intracranial blood flow are unclear.

RESPIRATORY AND MUSCLE CHANGES

Augmentation of breathing occurs upon standing; presumably, this causes a longer duration of negative intrathoracic pressure, preventing the easy collapse of the great veins. An increase in venous return to the heart results. At the same time, there is a rise in intra-abdominal pressure.[18]

The importance of peripheral skeletal muscle activity that occurs on standing ("the muscle pump") is unclear, but there is some contribution to enhanced venous return. This can be demonstrated by a fall in ankle venous pressure immediately upon standing, which presumably is caused by compression of superficial capacitance vessels by muscle contraction.[18]

REFERENCES

1. Gauer, OH: *Orthostatic hypotension: Closing remarks to Session I.* In Denolin, H and Demanet, JC (eds): *International symposium on neural control of the cardiovascular system and orthostatic regulation.* Cardiology 61[Suppl I]:91–92, 1976.
2. Reickert, H: *Die Physiologie der ortostatischen Regulation.* Cardiology 61[Suppl I]:69–77, 1976.
3. Borst, C, et al: *Mechanisms of initial heart rate response to postural change.* Am J Physiol 243:H676–H681, 1982.
4. Wieling, W, Dambrink, JHA, and Borst, C: *Cardiovascular effects of arising suddenly.* N Engl J Med 310:1189, 1984.
5. Berry, M: *Vascular clinics: Influences of position or arm and body in blood pressure determined by auscultation.* Proc Staff Meet Mayo Clin 16:29, 1961.

6. Hill, L: *The influence of the force of gravity on the circulation.* Lancet 1:338, 1985.
7. Brun, C, Knudsen, EOE, and Raaschou, F: *The influence of posture on the kidney function.* Acta Med Scand 122:332, 1945.
8. Sjostrand, T: *Uberdiebedeutung der lungen als blutdepot beim menschen.* Acta Physiol Scand 2:231, 1941.
9. Reid, JL: *Central and peripheral autonomic control mechanisms.* In Bannister, R (ed): *Autonomic Failure.* Oxford University Press, Oxford, 1983, pp 17–35.
10. Reis, DJ and Fuxe, K: *Adrenergic innervation of the carotid sinus.* Am J Physiol 215:1054–1057, 1968.
11. Bannister, R: *Degeneration of the autonomic nervous system.* Lancet II:175–179, 1971.
12. Bevegard, S: *In discussion of Reickert die Physiologie der ortostatischen Regulation.* Cardiology 61[Suppl I]:77, 1976.
13. Page, EB, et al: *Reflex venomotor activity in normal persons and in patients with postural hypotension.* Circulation 11:262–270, 1965.
14. Hollander, AP and Bouman, LN: *Cardiac acceleration in man elicited by a muscle–heart reflex.* J Appl Physiol 38:272–278, 1975.
15. Kirchheim, HR: *Systemic arterial baroreceptor reflexes.* Physiol Rev 56:100–176, 1976.
16. Marin Neto, JA, et al: *Mechanism of tachycardia on standing: Studies in normal individuals and in chronic Chagas' heart patients.* Cardiovasc Res 14:541–550, 1980.
17. Kopin, IJ, et al: *Urinary catecholamine metabolites distinguish different types of sympathetic neuronal dysfunction in patients with orthostatic hypotension.* J Clin Endocrinol Metab 57:632–637, 1983.
18. Newberry, PD, Hatch, AW, and Macdonald, JM: *Cardiorespiratory events preceding syncope induced by a combination of lower body negative pressure and head-up tilt.* Aerospace Medicine 41:373–378, 1970.
19. Guyton, AC: *Textbook of Medical Physiology,* ed 6. WB Saunders, Philadelphia, 1981, pp 232–245, 259–273.
20. Uhl, CR, et al: *Immunohistochemical mapping of enkephalin-containing cell bodies, fibres and nerve terminals in the brain stem of the rat.* Brain Res 167:77–91, 1979.

21. Laubie, M, et al: *Central cardiovascular effects of morphinometric peptides in dogs.* Eur J Pharmacol 46:67–71, 1977.

22. Schaz, K, et al: *Enkephalin effects on blood pressure, heart rate, and baroreceptor reflex.* Hypertension 2:395–407, 1980.

23. Share, L: *Role of cardiovascular receptors in the control of ADH release.* Cardiology 61[Suppl I]:51–64, 1976.

24. Fieschi, C and Bozzao, L: *Physiology of cerebral circulation.* In Carpi, A (ed): *Pharmacology of the Cerebral Circulation,* Vol I. Pergamon Press, Oxford, 1972, pp 1–33.

25. Thomas, DJ and Bannister, R: *Preservation of autoregulation of cerebral blood flow in autonomic failure.* J Neurol Sci 44:205–212, 1980.

26. Zijlstra, WG: *Cerebral metabolism.* In Minderhoud, JM (ed): *Cerebral Blood Flow: Basic Knowledge and Clinical Implications.* Excerpta Medica, Amsterdam, 1981, pp 55–78.

27. *Ibid,* pp 34–55.

28. Scheinberg, P and Stead, EA, Jr: *The cerebral blood flow in male subjects as measured by the nitrous oxide technique: Normal values for blood flow, oxygen utilization, glucose utilization and peripheral resistance, with observations on the effect of tilting and anxiety.* J Clin Invest 28:1163, 1949.

CHAPTER 2

ORTHOSTATIC HYPOTENSION DUE TO FUNCTIONAL DERANGEMENTS

INADEQUATE POSTURAL ADJUSTMENT

Asthenic Habitus With Poorly Developed Musculature

Physical Exertion

Bed Rest and/or Space Flight

Aging

Miscellaneous Causes

REDUCED EFFECTIVE CIRCULATORY BLOOD VOLUME

PHARMACOLOGIC AGENTS

MISCELLANEOUS CAUSES

Functional alterations in control of blood pressure (BP) on standing are the most common cause of postural hypotension and are usually transient (Table 2-1). Those homeostatic mechanisms that have been described in Chapter 1 may become impaired because of a wide variety of changes in both the internal and external milieu. In general, loss of adequate BP control is permanent only if the process affecting these mechanisms is caused by an organic disease.

TABLE 2-1. Functional Causes of Orthostatic Hypotension

Inadequate homeostatic mechanisms
- Inadequate postural adjustment
- Intense exercise
- Prolonged bed rest (?deconditioning)
- Space flight (?deconditioning)
- Aging
- Pregnancy
- Gastrectomy
- Anorexia nervosa
- Exposure to heat
- Marijuana use
- Fever

Reduced effective circulating blood volume
- Hemorrhage
- Dehydration
- Burns
- Diabetes insipidus
- Hemodialysis
- Peritoneal dialysis
- Large varicose veins
- Gravid uterus during last trimester

Pharmacologic agents
- Antihypertensives (any)
- Antipsychotics
- Antidepressants
- Vasodilators (nitrates, calcium-channel blockers)
- Narcotics
- Sedatives
- Antiparkinsonism drugs
- Alcohol
- Insulin

Miscellaneous
- Adrenal insufficiency (primary and secondary)
- Electrolyte derangement (hypokalemia, hypophosphatemia)
- Malignancy without metastases
- Infectious neuronitis (Guillain-Barré syndrome)
- Acute autonomic neuropathy

INADEQUATE POSTURAL ADJUSTMENT

Asthenic Habitus With Poorly Developed Musculature

Based on their considerable experience, Thomas and his colleagues[1] at the Mayo Clinic have described a group of individuals with a significant drop in systolic BP on standing, accompanied by an increase in diastolic BP and tachycardia. The consequent symptoms are suggestive of cerebral hypoxia. These individuals are usually of tall, asthenic habitus with poorly developed musculature.

The cardiovascular changes that occur in such patients consist of excessive pooling of blood in the distended capillary beds of the splanchnic and subpapillary skin plexuses. This leads to a decrease in effective blood volume and inadequate venous return, but an increase in peripheral vascular resistance. Presumably, excessive pooling of venous blood is the result of inadequate pumping from leg and arm muscles.

Physical Exertion

Following very vigorous exercise, often leading to exhaustion, orthostatic hypotension develops in otherwise normal subjects.[2] It is speculated that such extreme exertion results in marked peripheral vasodilatation either because of a direct effect of carbon dioxide accumulation or as a neural reflex.[3] There is apparently no relationship to the degree of physical fitness of the subject.

Bed Rest and/or Space Flight

Prolonged bed rest very commonly results in brief episodes of postural hypotension when the patient first stands. This is attributed to "deconditioning." The same mechanism may exist in astronauts after prolonged space flights; clear evidence exists that for a variable period after descent to earth orthostatic hypotension is a problem. Presumably, gravitational stresses leading to peripheral arterial and venous constriction need to be operating continually in order to ensure a prompt response to the upright posture. When there is a hiatus in such stimulation, such as with prolonged recumbency or space flight, some time is required before the homeostatic mechanisms function adequately.

Aging

In approximately one third of normal individuals over age 65, systolic BP declines by at least 20 mm Hg upon standing.[4,5] Diastolic BP and heart rate are largely unaffected.

Clinical expression of this orthostatic hypotension is variable; some patients complain of dizziness or syncope, but many have no symptoms. The pathophysiologic mechanisms responsible probably reflect a mosaic of causes, but baroreceptor reflex derangements are less common than in comparable younger subjects with orthostatic hypotension.[6] Robinson and his colleagues[6] showed minor reductions in supine plasma catecholamines in elderly subjects, but no differences in these levels from controls when measured upon standing. This finding suggested that sympathetic function was normal in their study group.[6] These data supported the earlier conclusions of Caird[5] and MacLennan[7] and their colleagues, as well as more recently accumulated evidence,[8] that orthostatic hypotension in the elderly is usually related to factors other than autonomic neuropathy.

Nevertheless, data that autonomic function *declines* with age are indisputable. R–R interval variability, dependent on parasympathetic integrity, decreases;[9] baroreceptor function in elderly hypertensives also is diminished.[10] Additionally, generalized neuronal loss,[11] decreased numbers of beta receptors[12] with reduced function,[13] and diminished responsiveness to catecholamines[14] have all been demonstrated.

Exacerbation of orthostatic hypotension after eating is prevalent in the elderly; Lipsitz and colleagues[15] recently showed significant reductions in postprandial BP in elderly nursing home subjects, some of whom had syncope. The mechanism is unclear; excessive pooling of blood in the splanchnic circulation may be responsible.[15]

Why some elderly subjects have dizziness and syncope while others do not remains puzzling, but data presented by Wollner and associates[16] suggest that there is a failure of cerebral autoregulation in some. These authors speculate that the sympathetic pathways that normally participate in cerebral vessel control may be impaired in some elderly patients.

Miscellaneous Causes

Peripheral pooling of blood occurs early during pregnancy, probably because of the direct action of hormones causing excessive dilatation of peripheral veins.[17] During the latter stages of pregnancy, however, the gravid uterus acts as a physical barrier to venous return by compression of the inferior vena cava.

Disturbances in postural regulation of BP are seen occasionally in patients who have had gastrectomy; the precise mechanism is unclear, but Thomas and colleagues[1] have suggested that in some way this operation impedes the return of venous blood to the heart. Obviously, another potential mechanism, particularly in those patients undergoing total gastrectomy, would be deficiency of intrinsic factor or folate leading to peripheral neuropathy, with subsequent impairment of peripheral vasoconstrictor function. This is discussed more fully in Chapter 3.

Postural hypotension has been reported in patients with severe forms of anorexia nervosa. The presumed pathogenesis in these patients is similar to that which has been postulated for individuals of tall, asthenic habitus: The poorly developed, or atrophic, peripheral musculature provides little or no "venous pump" for the return of blood to the thorax; this encourages marked pooling in the extremities. It has also been suggested that catecholamine release is deficient in this group.[18]

Merritt, Cook, and Davis[19] have reported orthostatic hypotension in three male subjects with glaucoma who were given Mexican marijuana cigarettes to smoke. Although previous studies indicated that blends of Mexican marijuanas and oral synthetic delta-9-tetrahydrocannabinol (THC) had produced sudden precipitous falls in systolic blood pressure,[20] this was the first demonstration that naturally occurring marijuana could cause significant hypotension. The precise mechanism is uncertain, but pretreatment with both propranolol and atropine can fully inhibit the effect of delta 9-THC on the cardiovascular system.[21]

Febrile patients often have orthostatic drops in BP. In a clinical experiment, 50 percent of normal individuals developed syncope when upright after 20 minutes of immersion in a 40°C bath.[22] One may speculate that this is due to a temporary unresponsiveness of peripheral arterioles to sympathetic constrictor influences. The same phenomenon probably occurs in Scandinavian sauna habitués who, after prolonged intense exposure to steam bathing, can immerse themselves into the icy cold water of the Gulf of Finland with no clinical signs of peripheral vasoconstriction or adverse effect.[23]

REDUCED EFFECTIVE CIRCULATORY BLOOD VOLUME

The maintenance of normal cardiac output and BP is dependent on both adequate peripheral vascular resistance and sufficient blood volume. When the filling pressure of the left ventricle falls below certain critical levels, not enough volume is available to stretch myocardial fibers during diastole, and therefore an inevitable reduction in output occurs. Any condition that leads to direct loss of blood or plasma from the circulation (hemorrhage, dehydration, burns, diabetes insipidus, hemodialysis, and peritoneal dialysis) may induce postural hypotension. The primary disease process is clinically apparent, and the orthostatic hypotension is a secondary phenomenon that clears when volume is restored.

Additionally, sequestration of blood in the extremities—as has been described with extensive varicose veins or because of obstruction of venous return by the gravid uterus during the last trimester of pregnancy—diminishes left ventricular filling pressure. The same mechanism probably occurs in patients with very large left-to-right cardiac shunts. Those undergoing hemodialysis are not only at risk for substantial, albeit temporary, reductions in volume; another problem in these patients is a lack of responsiveness of vascular smooth muscle to sympathetic stimulation, which occasionally occurs after dialysis. Further, patients with chronic renal failure may also have sympathetic nerve and baroreceptor dysfunction[24] (see Chapter 4).

PHARMACOLOGIC AGENTS

One of the most common causes of orthostatic hypotension is the ingestion of medication. The list of agents responsible is ubiquitous; in fact, virtually any compound that affects vascular tone, catecholamine homeostasis, or blood volume should be suspect until excluded. Obviously, antihypertensive drugs are important potential offenders. Medications that interfere with peripheral sympathetic activity such as guanethidine, rauwolfia derivatives, and phenothiazines may produce some degree of orthostasis. Drugs that reduce blood volume or change electrolyte concentrations in vascular smooth muscle, such as diuretics and calcium-channel blockers, also are suspect. Symptoms may occur with substances for which the hypotensive action is poorly understood (antidepressants, narcotics, and sedatives). Obviously, the direct dilating action of nitrates on peripheral arteries and veins may, with large enough doses, suppress reflex vascular constriction.

Although the chronic use of alcohol may lead to an irreversible autonomic neuropathy, Johnson[18] feels that there can be an initial toxic response without actual degeneration of autonomic nerves; with abstention from alcohol, full recovery may be expected. It is possible that this reflects a reversible disturbance of catecholamine release.[25]

Insulin use rarely causes temporary episodes of hypotension. The precise mechanism for this action is unclear, but it may be related to exaggerated displacement of fluid from the intravascular to the extravascular compartment, with resultant diminished effective circulating blood volume.[26] An alternative explanation is impairment of catecholamine responses, resulting in inadequate vasoconstriction. Studies have shown that the normal release of catecholamines and pancreatic polypeptide secondary to insulin injection is deficient in some patients with neurogenic orthostatic hypotension, probably as an early reflection of vagal neuropathy.[27–29]

MISCELLANEOUS CAUSES

Adrenal insufficiency results in deficient glucocorticoid and mineralocorticoid production. The consequent orthostatic hypotension, noted by Addison himself,[30] is the result of both a decrease in effective circulating plasma volume and a relative unresponsiveness of the vascular smooth muscle to circulating catecholamines.[31] Whether, as Cryer[31] suggests, there is also a defective baroreflex arc is a matter of conjecture. Hypotension usually is less severe in individuals with hypopituitarism because aldosterone secretion is partially preserved in such patients.

The orthostatic hypotension seen in patients with electrolyte disturbances is usually reversible.[3] The presumed mechanism is reduced responsiveness of peripheral arterial smooth muscle to sympathetic stimulation. It is known that changes in sodium–potassium flux in smooth muscle cells cause a variation in the degree of contractility, and that decreasing the amount of sodium ion in the smooth muscles renders peripheral arterioles less responsive to vasoconstrictive influences. A single case report of orthostatic hypotension in a patient with severe hypophosphatemia has appeared,[34] but the majority of those in whom postural BP control is temporarily defective have markedly depleted plasma potassium.

Occasionally, patients with panhypopituitarism or hypothyroidism may also have deficiencies in upright blood pressure maintenance, presumably again because of defective peripheral vasoconstriction or catecholamine utilization, or both.

Malignancies, particularly carcinoma without metastases, may create a reversible form of postural hypotension; symptoms and signs disappear with appropriate response of the tumor to therapy.[32] Additionally, of course, patients may develop permanent orthostatic hypotension secondary to both metastatic and nonmetastatic malignant syndromes (see Chapter 3).

Infectious neuronitis (principally the Guillain-Barré syndrome) is often associated with varying degrees of orthostatic hypotension. This is almost always reversible but may persist for as long as the autonomic neuropathy is present. The degree of autonomic failure is variable and is not directly related to the extent of sensory or motor involvement. Thus, some who require artificial respiration may have normal control of BP, yet others with severe autonomic dysfunction may demonstrate little or no motor or sensory loss.[18] The rare syndrome of acute autonomic neuropathy is probably a variant of infectious neuronitis, but only the autonomic nerves are affected. Orthostatic hypotension is often present in such patients.[33]

REFERENCES

1. Thomas, EJ, et al: *Orthostatic hypotension.* Mayo Clin Proc 56:117–125, 1981.
2. Eichna, LW, Horvath, SM, and Bean, WB: *Postexertional orthostatic hypotension.* Am J Med Sci 213:641, 1947.
3. Wagner, HN, Jr: *Orthostatic hypotension.* Bull Johns Hopkins Hosp 105:322–359, 1959.
4. Palmer, KT: *Studies into postural hypotension in elderly patients.* NJ Med J 96:43–45, 1983.
5. Caird, FI, Andrews, GR, and Kennedy, RD: *Effect of posture on blood pressure in the elderly.* Br Heart J 35:527–531, 1973.

6. Robinson, BJ, et al: *Do elderly patients with an excessive fall in blood pressure on standing have evidence of autonomic failure?* Clin Sci 64:587–591, 1983.

7. MacLennan, WJ, Hall, MRP, and Timothy, JI: *Postural hypotension in old age: Is it a disorder of the nervous system or of blood vessels?* Age Ageing 9:25–32, 1980.

8. Smith, SA and Fasler, JJ: *Age-related changes in autonomic function: Relationship with postural hypotension.* Age Ageing 12:206–210, 1983.

9. Smith, SE and Smith, SA: *Heart rate variability in healthy subjects measured with a bedside computer-based technique.* Clin Sci 61:379–383, 1981.

10. Bristow, JD, et al: *Diminished baroreflex sensitivity in high blood pressure in ageing man.* J Physiol (Lond) 1969; 202:45.

11. Collins, KJ: *Autonomic failure and the elderly.* In Bannister, R (ed): *Autonomic Failure.* Oxford University Press, Oxford, 1983, pp 489–507.

12. Schocken, DD and Roth, GS: *Reduced beta receptor concentration in aging man.* Nature 267:856–858, 1977.

13. Vestal, RE, Wood, AJJ, and Shand, DG: *Reduced beta adrenergic receptor sensitivity in the elderly.* Clin Pharmacol Ther 26:181–186, 1979.

14. Krall, JF, et al: *Age related elevation of plasma catecholamine concentration and reduced responsiveness of lymphocyte adenylate cyclase.* J Clin Endocrinol Metab 52:863–867, 1981.

15. Lipsitz, LA, et al: *Postprandial reduction in blood pressure in the elderly.* N Engl J Med 309:81–83, 1983.

16. Wollner, L, et al: *Failure of cerebral autoregulation as a cause of brain dysfunction in the elderly.* Br Med J 1:1117–1118, 1979.

17. Pyorala, T: *Cardiovascular response to the upright position during pregnancy.* Acta Obstet Gynecol Scand 45[Suppl]:5, 1966.

18. Johnson, RH: *Orthostatic hypotension in neurologic disease.* Cardiology 61[Suppl 1]:167, 1976.

19. Merritt, JC, Cook, CE, and David, KH: *Orthostatic hypotension after delta 9-tetrahydrocannabinol marihuana inhalation.* Ophthalmic Res 14:124–128, 1982.

20. Crawford, WJ, et al: *Tetrahydrocannabinol effect on elevated blood pressure in humans.* Prev Med 7:54, 1978.

21. Benowitz, NL, et al: *Cardiovascular effects of intravenous delta 9-tetrahydrocannabinol: Autonomic response mechanisms.* Clin Pharmacol Ther 25:440-446, 1979.

22. Horvat, SM and Botelho, SY: *Orthostatic hypotension following hot or cold baths.* J Appl Physiol 1:586–589, 1949.

23. Schatz, IJ: Personal observations.

24. Ewing, DJ and Willney, R: *Autonomic function in patients with chronic renal failure on intermittent hemodialysis.* Nephron 15:424–429, 1975.

25. Schenker, VJ, et al: *The effects of ethanol on amine metabolism in alcoholism.* In Maickel, P (ed): *Biochemical Factors in Alcoholism.* Pergamon Press, Oxford, 1967, p 39.

26. Mackay, JD, Hayakawa, H, and Watkins, PJ: *Cardiovascular effects of insulin: Plasma volume changes in diabetes.* Diabetologia 15:453–457, 1978.

27. Polinsky, RJ, et al: *Pancreatic polypeptide responses to hypoglycemia in chronic autonomic failure.* J Clin Endocrinol Metab 54:48–52, 1982.

28. McGrath, BP, et al: *Impaired pancreatic polypeptide release to insulin hypoglycemia in chronic autonomic failure with postural hypotension: Evidence for parasympathetic dysfunction.* Clin Sci 63:321–323, 1982.

29. Cryer, PE: *Disorders of sympathetic neural function in human diabetes mellitus: Hypoadrenergic and hyperadrenergic postural hypotension.* Metabolism 29:1186–1189, 1980.

30. *Collection of the Published Works of Addison.* New Sydenham Society, London, 1868, cited by Wagner, HN: *Orthostatic hypotension.* Bull Johns Hopkins Hosp 105:322–359, 1959.

31. Cryer, PE: *Mechanisms and management of postural hypotension.* In Cohen, MP and Foa, PP (eds): *Special Topics in Endocrinology and Metabolism,* Vol 1. Alan R Liss, New York, 1979, pp 79–91.

32. Siemson, JK and Meister, L: *Bronchogenic carcinoma associated with severe orthostatic hypotension.* Ann Intern Med 58:669–676, 1963.

33. Young, RR, et al: *Pure pan-dysautonomia with recovery.* Brain 98:613–635, 1975.

34. Nanji, AA and Freeman, HJ: *Postural hypotension and labile blood pressure associated with severe hypophosphatemia.* Int J Cardiol 5:379–381, 1984.

CHAPTER 3
ORTHOSTATIC HYPOTENSION DUE TO ORGANIC DERANGEMENTS

NEUROGENIC ORTHOSTATIC HYPOTENSION

Afferent Lesions

Central Disorders

IDIOPATHIC PARKINSONISM

RILEY-DAY SYNDROME (FAMILIAL DYSAUTONOMIA)

MISCELLANEOUS CAUSES

Efferent Defects

IDIOPATHIC ORTHOSTATIC HYPOTENSION

MULTIPLE-SYSTEM ATROPHY (SHY-DRAGER SYNDROME)

Clinical Description

Natural History

Pathology and Pathogenesis of Multiple-System Atrophy and Idiopathic Orthostatic Hypotension

Orthostatic Hypotension Associated With Excessive Sympathetic Discharge (Sympathicotonic Orthostatic Hypotension)

Orthostatic Hypotension and Mitral Valve Prolapse

Miscellaneous Lesions in the Spinal Cord

Disorders Primarily Affecting Sympathetic Chain and Postganglionic Nerves

DIABETES MELLITUS

MISCELLANEOUS NEUROPATHIES

DEFECTS IN PERIPHERAL VASCULATURE

Hyperbradykininism

Congenital Defect in Norepinephrine Release

There are three major pathophysiologic lesions leading to orthostatic hypotension: disorders of the central nervous system or the peripheral nerves, unresponsiveness of the vascular smooth muscle to sympathetic stimulation, and loss of effective circulating blood volume. Those conditions that are usually permanent or irreversible almost always fall within the first two of these categories; most individuals who have inadequate levels of effective circulating volume will respond to appropriate treatment.

The final common pathway for all of these disorders, of course, is low blood pressure (BP) upon standing, leading to cerebral hypoxia. Although the clinical presentation of dizziness, lightheadedness, or actual syncope upon standing may occur in most patients, other symptoms and signs differ substantially depending on the primary etiology. The natural course of these illnesses is also quite variable, ranging from an easily tolerable, relatively stable condition lasting many years to a progressive and serious deterioration in cardiovascular and neurologic function.

NEUROGENIC ORTHOSTATIC HYPOTENSION

Most chronic organic orthostatic hypotension is due to disorders of the central nervous system and the peripheral nerves. Obviously, these defects may occur whenever there is any substantial disturbance of the mechanisms described in Chapter 2. Tables 3-1, 3-2, and 3-3 list in detail the

TABLE 3-1. Neurogenic Orthostatic Hypotension

Lesions of the afferent limb of reflex arc, involving cranial nerves IX or X, or the baroreceptors
Diabetes mellitus
Alcohol
Holmes-Adie syndrome
Tabes dorsalis
Carotid sinus obliteration
Decreased baroreceptor sensitivity in hemodialysis patients

currently known neurologic disorders in which orthostatic hypotension may develop, and identify those parts of the reflex pathway that are affected.

Afferent Lesions

Lesions in the afferent limb of the reflex arc (baroreceptors, cranial nerves IX and X) are an uncommon cause of symptomatic orthostatic hypotension (see Table 3-1). Nevertheless, data from one series suggested that 23 percent of patients with diabetes mellitus and orthostatic hypotension have absent or defective circulatory reflexes associated with dysfunction in the afferent pathway.[1] It seems likely that in such patients the contribution of afferent limb defects to the production of orthostatic hypotension is obscured by

TABLE 3-2. Central Lesions

Idiopathic parkinsonism
Familial dysautonomia (Riley-Day syndrome)
Hydrocephalus
Parasellar tumors
Posterior fossa tumors
Posterior fossa surgery
Multiple cerebral infarcts
Wernicke's encephalopathy

TABLE 3-3. Efferent Lesions

A. Spinal cord and/or preganglionic nerves

- Idiopathic orthostatic hypotension
- Multiple-system atrophy
- Trauma
- Transverse myelitis
- Syringomyelia
- Intramedullary tumors
- Extramedullary tumors
- ?Sympathicotonic orthostatic hypotension (with or without mitral valve prolapse)

B. Postganglionic nerves

- Diabetes mellitus
- Chronic alcoholism
- Primary amyloidosis
- Chronic hemodialysis
- Tumors (nonmetastatic)
- Rheumatoid arthritis
- Porphyria
- Pernicious anemia
- Hansen's disease
- Tetanus
- Surgical sympathectomy
- Vincristine sulfate toxicity
- Perhexiline maleate toxicity
- Infectious neuronitis (reversible)
- Acute autonomic neuropathy (reversible)
- Vacor poisoning
- ?Chagas' disease
- ?Myasthenia gravis

the clinically more obvious symptoms and signs of motor and sensory neuropathy.

Persons with chronic alcoholism are said to have a lesion in the afferent part of the baroreceptor arc along with disorders elsewhere.[2] Rarer causes of orthostatic hypotension due to lesions in the afferent loop are tabes dorsalis,[1] the Holmes-Adie syndrome,[3] and obliteration of the carotid sinus by malignancy.[4]

Central Disorders

A number of disorders in the brain substance (see Table 3-2) may create autonomic dysfunction by disturbing those integrating structures necessary for the proper control of circulatory reflexes.

IDIOPATHIC PARKINSONISM

Autonomic dysfunction in a patient with Parkinson's disease was reported first in 1817 by James Parkinson himself.[5] Since then, reports based on anecdotal information have reflected the presence of orthostatic hypotension in parkinsonism. Not until the study of Gross, Bannister, and Godwin-Austen,[6] however, was a documented, controlled investigation made of the presence of orthostatic hypotension in Parkinson's disease. This demonstrated normal baroregulatory reflexes in the subjects with Parkinson's disease, but a substantial fall in BP on tilting when compared with the age-matched controls. The conclusion was that orthostatic hypotension in this group was the result of a central defect acting above the level of the medulla. When dysautonomia occurs in patients with parkinsonism, pathologic study has revealed concomitant loss of lateral horn cells but not to the same extent as one sees in patients with clear-cut multiple-system atrophy (Shy-Drager syndrome) (see below).

The introduction and use of L-dopa (levodopa) often unmask the presence of orthostatic hypotension in many patients with parkinsonism. Clearly, care must be taken to distinguish such patients from those with multiple-system atrophy. Although the cause of this orthostatic drop is unclear, there are several possibilities: physical inactivity, leading to peripheral muscle atrophy; the use of anticholinergic drugs; defective baroregulatory reflexes in the afferent, brain stem, or efferent pathways, causing inappropriate compensatory vasoconstriction; and, finally, decreased elasticity of the resistance vessels. Which of these possibilities is present, singly or in combination, is unknown, but it is likely that the most probable mechanism is related to a disorder of the nervous system above the level of the medulla, probably in the area of the substantia nigra, which in some way negatively influences circulatory homeostasis.

It should be emphasized nonetheless that during the initial stages of the illness, patients with the Shy-Drager syndrome may show signs only of extrapyramidal deficits and orthostatic hypotension. In such clinical situations, the easy conclusion is that the patient suffers from idiopathic parkinsonism with associated postural BP defects. It is not until later that the more diffuse nature of the neurologic disorder becomes apparent and, with it, the more ominous prognosis of multiple-system atrophy must be recognized.

RILEY-DAY SYNDROME (FAMILIAL DYSAUTONOMIA)

This rare disorder, the Riley-Day syndrome, results in central baroreceptor reflex failure. It is characterized by orthostatic hypotension, autonomic instability, impaired taste and lacrimation, diminished pain and temperature sensation, frequent pneumonia, gastrointestinal disturbances, and early death. It is transmitted as an autosomal recessive gene with a frequency among Ashkenazi Jews of about 1 percent, and an incidence in the same population of one in 20,000. Sephardic Jews are spared. Those who do survive into adulthood have a propensity toward sudden death, estimated at 25 percent in one series.[7]

MISCELLANEOUS CAUSES

Cerebral malformations, including hydrocephalus, have also been occasionally accompanied by autonomic failure.[8]

Brain tumors that interfere with or impinge on reflex connections may often be accompanied by variable signs of autonomic disturbances, with the principal manifestation being orthostatic hypotension;[9] such lesions include craniopharyngioma.[10] In fact, orthostatic hypotension may be a major clinical manifestation of tumors of the posterior fossa.[9]

Damage to integrating centers that occurs during neurosurgical procedures may also induce orthostatic hypotension. Patients with multiple cerebral infarcts[11] and Wernicke's encephalopathy[12–14] often develop defects in autonomic reflex control of the BP. Birchfield[13] found that 32 of 40 patients with Wernicke's disease had orthostatic hypotension, although most were asymptomatic. The site of the autonomic defect in this disorder may be at one or more of several levels, since the hypothalamus, midbrain, tegmentum, and fourth ventricle roof nuclei are consistently involved.[14]

Efferent Defects

Major interest in orthostatic hypotension as a separate clinical syndrome first started with the seminal report of Bradbury and Eggleston[15] in 1925. Prior to that time, a number of anecdotal case reports had appeared, as an almost certain reflection of the fact that physicians interested in the subject had assessed and catalogued patients with orthostatic hypotension. Wagner,[16] in his comprehensive review of this subject, cites several observers, beginning in the early 19th century, who very likely recorded instances of orthostatic hypotension. Bradbury and Eggleston probably described patients who had neurogenic orthostatic hypotension of several different causes. Since then, the classification has become more sophisticated. At present, neurogenic orthostatic hypotension may be conveniently divided into those circulatory disturbances secondary to a clearly recognized underlying neurologic disease (for instance, brain tumors, syringomyelia, trauma, polyneuropathy) and those in whom an underlying, identifiable lesion is not apparent.

In 1960, Shy and Drager[17] described the clinical and pathologic findings in two patients, each of whom had severe orthostatic hypotension. At first, it was felt that this report was merely a variant of what previously had been considered idiopathic orthostatic hypotension, but subsequently this was shown not to be the case.[18] It has become apparent, however, that the Shy-Drager syndrome is distinct and separate from other organic causes of orthostatic hypotension (Table 3-4).

TABLE 3-4. Differential Diagnosis of Major Forms of Neurogenic Orthostatic Hypotension

	Multiple-system atrophy (Shy-Drager syndrome)	Idiopathic orthostatic hypotension	Idiopathic parkinsonism	Sympathicotonic orthostatic hypotension
Presenting symptoms and signs	Orthostatic hypotension, severity variable; incontinence or impotence; diffuse CNS deficits	Orthostatic hypotension, severity variable; incontinence; impotence; anhidrosis	Orthostatic hypotension (generally not severe, often superimposed on clearcut signs and symptoms of parkinsonism; may be aggravated by levodopa)	Orthostatic hypotension, often mild; associated complaints of palpitations; fatigue, chest pain; evidence of mitral valve prolapse in some
Neurologic manifestations	Signs and symptoms of severely progressive pyramidal and extrapyramidal involvement, as well as cerebellar degeneration and autonomic failure	Some progression of signs associated with autonomic degeneration: anhidrosis, impotence, sphincter disturbances	Signs and symptoms of extrapyramidal involvement; dementia in some	No significant findings

Early differential diagnostic signs	Normal plasma levels of norepinephrine while recumbent, with only a slight rise on standing (compared with threefold rise in normal subjects)	Very low plasma norepinephrine levels while recumbent, may have no increase on standing. Patients supersensitive to norepinephrine infusion, with dramatic rise in blood pressure in response to a very small amount (indicating that postsynaptic neurons are affected)	Numerous evaluations over many months to assess disease progression are required to rule out Shy-Drager syndrome and idiopathic orthostatic hypotension. Orthostatic symptoms do not get worse with time.	Excessive chronotropic response to standing (>25 beats/minute), associated with signs of sympathetic overactivity (pallor, sweating). Normal norepinephrine response to standing
Prognosis	Usually fatal within 7–8 years of diagnosis; death results from inanition or pneumonia	Usually manageable with physical or drug treatment	Orthostatic hypotension is pharmacologically manageable	Beta-adrenergic blocker therapy usually successful

The term multiple-system atrophy is now used as a more accurate reflection of the diffuse nature of the pathologic lesion in the disease originally described by Shy and Drager.[19]

IDIOPATHIC ORTHOSTATIC HYPOTENSION

Idiopathic orthostatic hypotension is a primary form of orthostatic hypotension in which repeated attempts to demonstrate a specific neurologic cause have been fruitless; it has been termed progressive autonomic failure by some workers.[20] Men are much more commonly affected than women (4:1 or 5:1). The onset is slow and insidious; upon close questioning, the patient often recalls that symptoms first came on several years before initially seeking advice from a physician. Complaints may be unsteadiness, or dizziness, or actual faintness upon standing, almost always worse in the morning, or sometimes after meals. In men, advice is often sought from the urologist, because of symptoms of bladder sphincter disturbance. Actual incontinence may be present. Very gradually, symptoms of other forms of autonomic disturbance occur, such as impotency, loss of libido, and inability to achieve and maintain erection, to ejaculate, and to appreciate orgasm. Retrograde ejaculation frequently occurs. In women, urinary retention or incontinence is also a frequent early symptom. Signs of sympathetic and parasympathetic activity, such as nausea, pallor, and cold perspiration, are absent or diminished, since they require normal autonomic function.

Progression of orthostatic hypotension is variable. Many persons go on to develop signs of other neurologic deficits, clearly indicating multiple-system atrophy (see below). In the remainder, no evidence of new central nervous system (CNS) defects are apparent, even though postural hypotension may become more severe. However, Johnson[21] states he has followed a group of patients with idiopathic orthostatic hypotension who have shown no worsening of defective BP control, and no progression of peripheral autonomic deficiency, for as long as 12 to 15 years. Others agree.[22]

MULTIPLE-SYSTEM ATROPHY (SHY-DRAGER SYNDROME)

In 1960, Milton Shy and Glenn Drager, at the National Institutes of Health, described the clinical findings in two patients with orthostatic hypotension, and the results of a carefully performed autopsy in one.[17]

The following characteristics (see Table 3-4) were observed: orthostatic hypotension, urinary and rectal incontinence, loss of sweating, iris atrophy, external ocular palsies, rigidity, tremor, loss of associated movements, impotence, atonic bladder and loss of rectal sphincter tone, fasciculations, wasting of distal muscles, evidence of a neuropathic lesion in the electromyogram that suggested involvement of the anterior horn cells, and the presence of a neuropathic lesion in the muscle biopsy. The age of onset was between the fifth and seventh decades, and hypotension was a relatively late finding.

Clinical Description

The above description by Shy and Drager has been confirmed by many others. Bannister[19] has suggested that the more descriptive term multiple-system atrophy be used. Thomas and colleagues[22] from the Mayo Clinic have had extensive experience with patients referred to that institution and have expanded the observations of Shy and Drager. They point out that there is a conspicuous involvement of central motor tracts including the corticobulbar, corticospinal, extrapyramidal, and cerebellar systems. Patients may demonstrate variable defects, but a parkinsonian-like syndrome is most apparent. It follows, therefore, that when a patient presents with both parkinsonism and orthostatic hypotension, an important clinical distinction must be made among multiple-system atrophy, idiopathic orthostatic hypotension, and idiopathic parkinsonism with associated hypotension. A meticulous search for signs and symptoms of diffuse CNS disease is necessary; in the absence of such findings, multiple-system atrophy may be excluded for the time being. Subsequently, the distinction between idiopathic parkinsonism with associated hypotension and idiopathic orthostatic hypotension becomes clear on the basis of clinical characteristics: patients with idiopathic orthostatic hypotension have postural hypotension as their predominant sign, usually accompanied by indications of sphincter disturbance and loss of sympathetic function, but with minor degrees of parkinsonism-like features.

In multiple-system atrophy, the sensory systems are not involved, and dementia is not apparent. Patients retain intellectual faculties even during the most debilitating phases of their illness. This is in contrast to the mental impairment often seen in other diffuse neurologic diseases. The two patients in Shy and Drager's original report had iris atrophy, but none of the 57 patients in the Mayo Clinic group demonstrated this finding.[34] Pupillary abnormalities and Horner's syndrome are often present and include alternating anisocoria and abnormal responses to drugs.[23] Lower motor neuron involvement manifested by atrophy and fasciculations and a lax anal sphincter are present frequently; electromyography of the sphincter muscle demonstrates denervation potentials.[22]

Cholinergic dysfunction is occasionally present, and may reflect vagal, ocular, bladder, and sweat-gland disturbances.[24–26] Khurana and coworkers[24] observed that severe constipation was the initial symptom in their patients, followed subsequently by diffuse autonomic neuropathic complaints.

Several types of breathing disturbance occur in patients with multiple-system atrophy. The most common of these has been the obstructive sleep apnea syndrome.[27–30] This may be central, with no respiratory motor activity, or obstructive, where there is disturbance of pharyngeal and laryngeal muscles. Brain stem sensitivity to carbon dioxide concentration may be altered.[30] Apnea sometimes occurs when the patient is awake; such patients may have involuntary gasps or so-called "cluster" breathing.[31] Sinus arrhythmia during sleep is blunted; it is suggested that a "decoupling" of heart rate from the respiratory cycle occurs in these patients.

One of the more common—albeit generally unrecognized—signs in multiple-system atrophy is laryngeal stridor. Gradual and insidious hoarseness develops; often, the process is so slow that the patient and family are unaware of its presence during its initial stages. Actual stridor becomes apparent during the later stages of the disease. Examination by laryngoscopy reveals laryngeal abductor paresis; the cords may appear to be immobile.[32]

Hanson, Ludlow, and Bassick[33] reported 11 of 12 patients with multiple-system atrophy had laryngeal movement disorders. Vocal impairment presented as a breathy and strained voice with reduced loudness. In comparison with control patients, the group with multiple-system atrophy had excessive hoarseness and a slow and deliberate speaking rate; these were considered distinguishing features. These authors conclude that the laryngeal pathology specifically points to brain stem disease.

Natural History

The most detailed information about the natural history of multiple-system atrophy is available from the Mayo Clinic.[34] Although Thomas and Schirger reported on "57 neurologically affected patients . . . with idiopathic orthostatic hypotension," a review of their criteria for selection suggests that most had signs of diffuse CNS disease. It is likely that the majority would now be classified as having multiple-system atrophy, as differentiated from idiopathic orthostatic hypotension. These data, as well as others, suggest that there is a gradual evolution of symptoms and signs and a slowly progressive deterioration in each patient. Precise predictions about the course of the illness, however, are impossible. In some, bladder and anal sphincter disturbances, and impotence may appear initially, whereas orthostatic hypotension with or without other neurologic complaints may not occur for several years. Conversely, hypotension may create the initial complaints; only gradually do signs of both central and peripheral neurologic disorders become apparent. Rather marked disability may be produced, therefore, by any one of the major manifestations of this illness; a patient may be substantially impaired because of hypotension and yet show only minor neurologic deficits or, conversely, may have very severe neurologic disturbance with only a modest, relatively well-tolerated decline in BP upon standing.

Thomas and Schirger's study indicated that death occurred on the average 7 to 8 years after the symptomatic onset of the disease, and 4 to 5 years after first neurologic signs appeared. Occasional patients, nonetheless, may have a more indolent course, with survival of 10 and sometimes 15 years from the onset of symptoms.[4]

Pathology and Pathogenesis of Multiple-System Atrophy and Idiopathic Orthostatic Hypotension

The original report by Shy and Drager[17] pointed out the diffuse nature of the pathologic process, with histologic evidence of degeneration in the autonomic nervous system, the corticobulbar and corticospinal tracts, some of the basal ganglia, and portions of the cerebellar system. Although initial speculation was that some of these changes might be secondary to chronic hypoxia from hypotension, this was subsequently shown not to be true.[18] Other studies of the neuropathologic changes confirmed Shy and Drager's observations, and expanded upon them.[35–40] It became apparent that two distinct patient groups emerged: those with autonomic failure plus parkinsonism but without other neurologic lesions, and those with diffuse neurologic changes.

Furthermore, a clinical correlation can be made that supports such a distinction: The patients with idiopathic orthostatic hypotension have autonomic failure and symptoms and signs of parkinsonism without further neurologic disturbance. Patients with multiple-system atrophy have additional diffuse neurologic signs and symptoms. In both groups, the loss of pigmented cells in the substantia nigra clearly relates to the presence of clinical parkinsonism; cell counting shows similar degrees of intermediolateral cell loss in both.

Other pathologic changes noted, in addition to striatonigral cell loss, include occasional cytoplasmic inclusion bodies in pigmented neurons. Characteristic of multiple-system atrophy, however, is the loss of cells in systems other than the basal ganglia and intermediolateral columns[40] (Fig. 3-1). Histologic overlap with other atrophic disorders is common.

As described above, a particular finding in patients with multiple-system atrophy is the presence of severe selective atrophy of the cricoarytenoid muscles, which are the sole abductors of the vocal cord, resulting in clinical laryngeal stridor. In two patients described, the changes were mainly myopathic, but in two other cases, there were definite signs of denervation atrophy.[32]

The pathogenesis of both idiopathic orthostatic hypotension and multiple-system atrophy is uncertain; no known metabolic, infectious, or provoking factors have been identified as yet. Sporadic reports about the familial occurrence of multiple-system atrophy have appeared,[41] but in general, there seem to be no familial tendencies. A recent study, however, does suggest that there may be a genetic predisposition to idiopathic orthostatic hypotension. Bannister, Mawbray, and Sidgwick[42] found that the frequency of HLA antigen Aw32 was 13 times more common in patients with idiopathic orthostatic hypotension than in controls. They speculated that a genetic predisposition to the disease might lead to a defect in catecholamine metabolism in the brain, or might possibly affect the immune response to a virus. Since some patients with idiopathic orthostatic hypotension develop hyaline eosinophilic cytoplasmic neuronal inclusions (Lewy bodies) in the brain stem, and the pathologic features of idiopathic orthostatic hypotension include degeneration of pigmented catecholamine-containing cells in the brain stem and cholinergic cells in the intermediolateral columns, these changes might be interpreted as reflecting a genetic metabolic defect. Perhaps idiopathic orthostatic hypotension is the result of a genetically determined biochemical flaw in cerebral catecholamine metabolism, and this gene lies within the HLA region. The strong association with an A-locus antigen might make this more likely than an immunologic cause of the syndrome.[42]

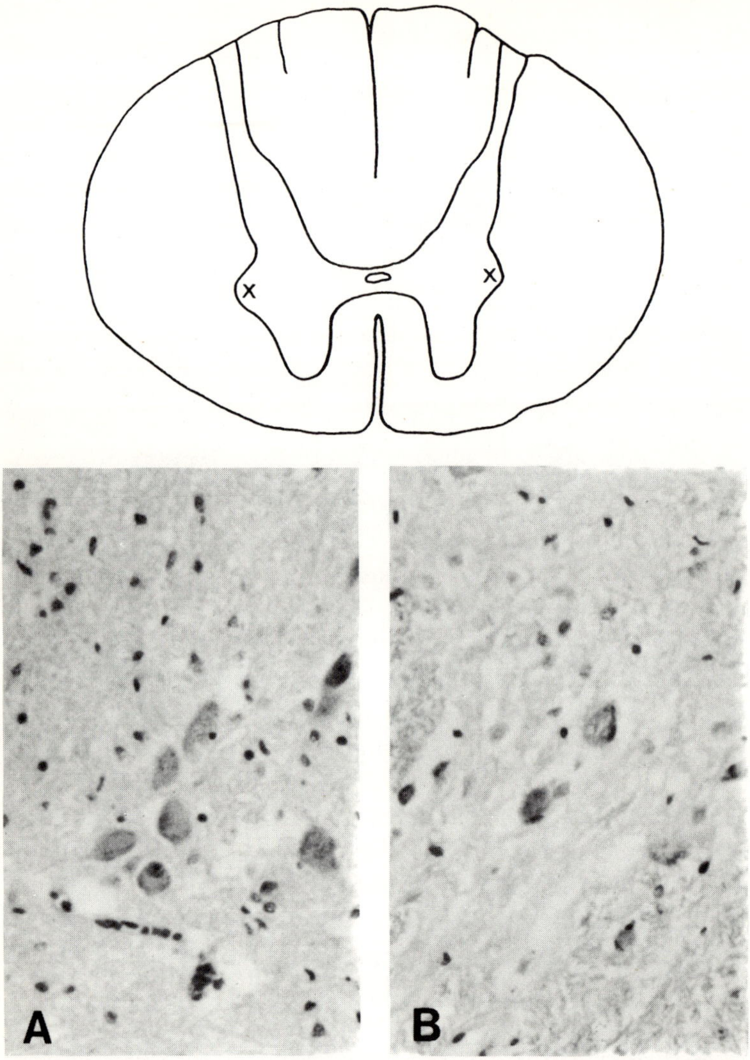

FIGURE 3-1. (*Top*) Upper thoracic spinal cord. Each intermediolateral nucleus is marked by an "x". (*Bottom*) Intermediolateral nucleus of upper thoracic spinal cord (Hematoxylin and eosin stain, original magnification × 170). (*A*) Normal; (*B*) Multiple-system atrophy. Note marked depletion of neurons compared with normal in *A*. (Photomicrographs courtesy of Dr. John Hardman.)

There also is a need to identify the lesions responsible for autonomic failure. Oppenheimer[38] points out that nerve cells, although in good health, may be unable to function normally because of a biochemical defect—as apparently occurs with striatal nerves in Parkinson's disease. When selective neuronal structures degenerate, is this due to a common biochemical property of the cell?

Further questions about the precise classification of these patients will continue to exist until specific neuropathologic distinction among idiopathic parkinsonism, multiple-system atrophy, and idiopathic orthostatic hypotension is possible in most cases.

As Polinsky has pointed out, the ultimate pathophysiologic expression of autonomic nervous system disease is multiple: deficient baroreceptor modulation, supersensitivity of adrenergic receptors, probable beta-adrenergic dysfunction, and vagal disorder. The major manifestation of these disturbances usually is orthostatic hypotension, although other clinical symptoms and signs may also appear.

Orthostatic Hypotension Associated With Excessive Sympathetic Discharge (Sympathicotonic Orthostatic Hypotension)

Forms of orthostatic hypotension in which symptoms appear because of a decrease in systolic BP but an *excessive* tachycardia have been described.[43] This has been called "hypersympathicotonic orthostatic hypotension";[44,45] adequate data on the prevalence of this form of postural defect are unavailable, but Demanet[44] found 10 of 21 patients who were referred to him for "spontaneously occurring orthostatic hypotension" whom he considered to have this disorder.

Generally, exaggerated sympathetic reflexes with excessive orthostatic tachycardia accompanying the orthostatic hypotension are its hallmarks.[45] Other signs of increased sympathetic discharge, such as pallor and sweating, also appear.

The pathophysiologic basis for this condition may consist of decreased alpha-adrenergic and normal beta-adrenergic responses. Polinsky and associates[46] studied a group of patients with sympathicotonic orthostatic hypotension and found they had normal basal levels of norepinephrine, and low mean BP when reclining. During infusions of norepinephrine, however, there was a less-than-normal rise in the mean BP when compared with controls. In addition, they had a normal pressor response to the infusion of tyramine. It was concluded that the tachycardia reflected an excessive response of the beta-sympathetic receptors to standing; however, the normal (or slightly subnormal) response to different types of exogenous pressors indicated an impaired effector organ response.[46]

Another view of sympathicotonic orthostatic hypotension has been presented by Cryer, who has observed a similar clinical form of orthostatic hypotension in patients with diabetes mellitus; he feels that in this group it is caused by a sharply reduced red blood cell mass producing a decrease in effective intravascular volume.[47]

Orthostatic Hypotension and Mitral Valve Prolapse

Autonomic dysfunction occurs in substantial numbers of patients with prolapse of the mitral valve[48–50] (Table 3-5). Often this is manifested by a significant decline in systolic BP, and an excessive tachycardia on standing. Accompanying symptoms of dizziness, palpitations, and fatigue are common.

Wooley makes the interesting suggestion that a number of previously described cardiac disorders in which fatigue, cardiovascular irritability, and vague symptoms occurred ("irritable heart"—J.M. DaCosta, 1864; "soldier's heart"—Thomas Lewis, James MacKenzie, 1916–1940; "neurocirculatory asthenia"—P.D. White, M. Cohen, 1931–1972) all may be forms of autonomic instability in which mitral valve prolapse may be one—but not the only—physical sign.[51] Gaffney and coworkers provide strong data to support this

TABLE 3-5. Evidence for Autonomic Dysfunction in Patients with Mitral Valve Prolapse

	Adrenergic tone	Parasympathetic tone
Gaffney et al[50]	Increased alpha Normal beta	Decreased
Boudoulas et al[53]	Increased (as measured by urinary and plasma catecholamine)	—
Coghlan[54]	—	Increased? (exaggerated bradycardia during Valsalva maneuver)

thesis, showing decreased parasympathetic but increased alpha- and normal beta-adrenergic tone and responsiveness in women with mitral prolapse.[50] The same workers subsequently demonstrated that in symptomatic patients with mitral valve prolapse two distinct subgroups emerged: those with normal heart rates but increased vasoconstriction, and those with orthostatic tachycardia. In the former, reduced cardiac output and marked vasoconstriction were observed.[52]

Boudoulas and coworkers[53] found excessive adrenergic tone, as measured by urinary and plasma catecholamines in their patients with mitral valve prolapse, all of whom were symptomatic. Other data demonstrated erratic autonomic cardiovascular control, and, in particular, exaggerated bradycardia during the recovery phase of the Valsalva maneuver.[54]

As might be expected during the early stages of investigation of autonomic dysfunction in this syndrome, different interpretations are provided. James and his group from Alabama[54] question whether excessive alpha responsiveness and diminished vagal tone exist; instead they agree with others[55] that abnormal forebrain modulation of the baroreceptor reflex may operate in these subjects, inducing excessive bradycardia. The matter of excessive orthostatic tachycardia remains unanswered, however.

Clearly, further intensive study of the relationship between mitral valve prolapse and autonomic dysfunction are warranted.

Miscellaneous Lesions in the Spinal Cord

A number of uncommon disorders that affect intermediolateral column function produce autonomic failure and subsequent orthostatic hypotension. These include direct trauma to the spinal cord, producing quadriplegia,[57] transverse myelitis, syringomyelia, and various intramedullary and extramedullary tumors. The presence of the primary lesion is usually quite apparent.

Disorders Primarily Affecting Sympathetic Chain and Postganglionic Nerves

DIABETES MELLITUS

Orthostatic hypotension is an important and disabling complication in patients with diabetic neuropathy. The lesion most likely responsible is damage to the sympathetic vasoconstrictor nerves.[58] Nevertheless, some patients with diabetes mellitus may have postural hypotension associated with an exaggerated sympathetic response; this is probably a form of sympathicotonic orthostatic hypotension (see above). Whether this is antecedent to the development of sympathetic vasoconstrictor deficiency is unclear. Hypotension may also be aggravated by insulin injection, perhaps because of displacement of fluid from intravascular to extravascular compartments.[59] Polinsky and others[60] have demonstrated that there is an impaired catecholamine and pancreatic polypeptide response to insulin-induced hypoglycemia. Although their studies were performed in patients with autonomic dysfunction due to multiple-system atrophy and idiopathic orthostatic hypotension, the assumption that the same mechanism may exist in those with diabetic neuropathy would appear to be acceptable. Since pancreatic polypeptide release during hypoglycemia is independent of the sympathoadrenal medullary response, and because such release is abolished by truncal vagotomy and unaffected by splanchnic nerve section, it is possible that the autonomic dysfunction involves both the parasympathetic and the sympathetic nervous systems in such patients. In fact, data are available that clearly point to vagal impairment in some.[61]

Evidence of autonomic neuropathy usually is present in patients with diabetes mellitus well before overt clinical signs of hypotension appear. Moorhouse, Carter, and Doupe[62] first demonstrated conclusively that diminished sympathetic vasoconstrictor tone was responsible for the abnormal vascular responses in diabetic neuropathy. Since then, a number of investigators have shown that sympathetic and parasympathetic dysfunction is common;[63–66] the techniques used have included measuring the beat-to-beat variation in heart rate, the response to the Valsalva maneuver, orthostatic heart rate variations, and sustained hand grip.

Cryer and colleagues have provided human experimental evidence that suggests the site of the sympathetic lesion in these patients is in the postganglionic neurons, as is seen in idiopathic orthostatic hypotension.[67]

It is apparent, however, that autonomic neuropathy has little or no effect on the metabolic responses of diabetic patients to exercise and to changes in blood glucose level, although the cardiovascular system has an increased sensitivity to circulating catecholamines in those with autonomic neuropathy. Hilsted[58] speculates that autonomic and somatic neuropathy may develop in tandem and may progress at the same rate in the parasympathetic and sympathetic systems as well as in the preganglionic and postganglionic neurons.

MISCELLANEOUS NEUROPATHIES

Virtually any peripheral neuropathy may interfere sufficiently with peripheral vasoconstrictor nerve function to create orthostatic hypotension.

Persons with chronic alcoholism may develop postural defects in BP control; the lesions in such patients are likely located both in the afferent and efferent parts of the reflex arc. Autonomic ganglionic cell dysfunction may occur,[63] and overall catecholamine production sometimes is diminished.[68]

Patients with primary amyloidosis manifest a form of orthostatic hypotension that is particularly resistant to therapy and markedly progressive in nature. This is caused by direct amyloid infiltration of peripheral nerves, including the sympathetic chain.[69] Perhaps 15 percent of all patients with primary amyloidosis will develop autonomic neuropathy, although the extent to which this produces postural symptoms is unclear. Nevertheless, Kelly and associates[70] reported that 42 percent of their patients with amyloid neuropathy had orthostatic hypotension as a major disability. Occasionally, symptoms of orthostatic hypotension may precede other manifestations of amyloidosis or, rarely, may be the sole sign of the disease.

The association of acute intermittent porphyria with orthostatic hypotension has been described.[71] A less rare phenomenon is the presence of postural hypotension in patients with malignancy;[72] if no metastases exist, then orthostatic hypotension sometimes disappears after successful eradication of the primary tumor. Other possible pathogenetic mechanisms in those with metastatic disease consist of diffuse polyneuropathy, and direct extension of a head and neck tumor into the carotid sinus.[86]

Patients with chronic renal failure, particularly those undergoing chronic hemodialysis, develop orthostatic hypotension with some frequency. Sweat dysfunction in this group was first demonstrated in 1968;[73] subsequently, Ewing and Willney showed that 50 percent of such patients have abnormal responses to testing of autonomic function.[74] It is unclear which part of the reflex arc is involved; in fact, it has been suggested that the efferent sympathetic pathways may be intact in some patients on chronic hemodialysis.[75] Nies and colleagues demonstrated intact efferent sympathetic nerve function in five chronic patients who had hypotension during dialysis; their data indicated a probable defect in baroreceptor sensitivity.[76] Nevertheless, patients with chronic renal failure do develop uremic neuropathy, which may be the cause of postural hypotension.

The occurrence of orthostatic hypotension in pernicious anemia was first documented in 1962.[77] A later report confirmed this finding; the authors speculated that autonomic neuropathy caused the defect.[78] A recent study, however, demonstrated deficient catecholamine response in a patient with this syndrome.[79]

Clear-cut evidence of autonomic neuropathy was present in 9 of 18 patients with rheumatoid arthritis.[80] In some, orthostatic hypotension was the principal manifestation. The etiology is unclear, but since peripheral neuropathy in rheumatoid arthritis is believed to be caused by vasculitis, the same mechanism may exist when disease of the autonomic nerves is apparent. Obviously, amyloidosis may have developed in some.

Agents that interfere with adrenergic function, such as vincristine sulfate or perhexiline maleate when used therapeutically,[81,82] or the rodenticide vacor,[83] when exposed accidentally, may cause severe orthostatic hypotension.

Although patients with Chagas' disease are reported occasionally to develop autonomic dysfunction, it is unclear whether postural hypotension ever becomes a manifestation.[84] Similarly, a single report of the occurrence of orthostatic hypotension in a patient with myasthenia gravis has appeared; the significance, if any, of this association is unknown.[85]

DEFECTS IN PERIPHERAL VASCULATURE

Hyperbradykininism

A much rarer but better defined syndrome is that described by Streetin and coworkers in 1972.[56] These patients have excessive amounts of the endogenous vasodilator bradykinin. This substance causes arteriolar and venular dilatation. Under normal circumstances, it is inactivated by an enzyme, but rarely it may be deficient in quantity. Consequently, excessive amounts of the vasodilator circulate, producing orthostatic hypotension. Investigation of these patients suggest that sympathetic function is normal.

Congenital Defect in Norepinephrine Release

Careful study of a 33-year-old patient with severe orthostatic hypotension since the age of 2 and no stigmata of familial dysautonomia or neurologic disease disclosed very low levels of recumbent and upright plasma norepinephrine. In contrast, plasma epinephrine was normal, but plasma dopamine was elevated.[87]

Other data supported a diagnosis of a congenital defect in norepinephrine release, with elevated levels of dopamine and intact parasympathetic function.

REFERENCES

1. Sharpey-Schafer, EP and Taylor, PJ: *Absent circulatory reflexes in diabetic neuritis.* Lancet 1:559–562, 1960.
2. Barraclough, MA and Sharpey-Schafer, EP: *Hypotension from absent circulatory reflexes: Effects of alcohol, barbiturates, psychotherapeutic drugs and other mechanisms.* Lancet 1:1121–1126, 1963.
3. Johnson, RH, McLellan, DL, and Love, DR: *Orthostatic hypotension and the Holmes-Adie syndrome.* J Neurol Neurosurg Psychiatry 34:562–570, 1971.
4. Schatz, IJ: Unpublished observations.
5. Rajput, AH and Rozdilsky, B: *Dysautonomia in Parkinsonism: A clinicopathological study.* J Neurol Neurosurg Psychiatry 39:1092–1100, 1976.
6. Gross, M, Bannister, R, and Godwin-Austen, R: *Orthostatic hypotension in Parkinson's disease.* Lancet 1:174–176, 1972.
7. Dancis, J: *Familial dysautonomia.* In Bannister, R (ed): *Autonomic Failure.* Oxford University Press, Oxford, 1983, pp 615–639.

8. Appenzeller, O, Synder, R, and Kornfeld, M: *Autonomic failure in hydroencephaly.* J Neurol Neurosurg Psychiatry 33:532–543, 1970.

9. O'Malley, WE, O'Dougherty, DS, and Auth, TL: *Orthostatic hypotension as manifestation of posterior fossa tumor.* Dis Nerv Syst 31:846–850, 1970.

10. Thomas, JE, et al: *Orthostatic hypotension as a presenting sign in craniopharyngioma.* Neurol 11:418–423, 1961.

11. Hammarstrom, S and Lindgren, AGH: *Postural hypotension in a patient with multiple encephalomalacias.* Acta Med Scand 111:537–554, 1942.

12. Gravallese, MA, Jr and Victor, M: *Circulatory studies in Wernicke's encephalopathy: With special reference to the occurrence of a state of high cardiac output and postural hypotension.* Circulation 15:836–844, 1957.

13. Birchfield, RI: *Postural hypotension in Wernicke's disease.* Am J Med 3:404–414, 1964.

14. Cravioto, H, Kovsin, J, and Silberman, J: *Wernicke's encephalopathy.* Arch Neurol 4:510, 1961.

15. Bradbury, S and Eggleston, C: *Postural hypotension: A report of three cases.* Am Heart J 1:73–86, 1925.

16. Wagner, HN: *Orthostatic hypotension.* Bull Johns Hopkins Hosp 105:322–359, 1959.

17. Shy, DM and Drager, GA: *A neurological syndrome associated with orthostatic hypotension: A clinical-pathologic study.* Arch Neurol 2:511–527, 1960.

18. Schatz, IJ, Podolsky, S, and Frame, B: *Idiopathic orthostatic hypotension: Diagnosis and treatment.* JAMA 186:537–540, 1963.

19. Bannister, R: *Chronic autonomic failure with postural hypotension.* Lancet 2:404–406, 1979.

20. Bannister, R: *Treatment of progressive autonomic failure.* In Bannister, R (ed): *Autonomic Failure.* Oxford University Press, Oxford, 1983, pp 316–334.

21. Johnson, RH: In discussion of Schirger, A and Thomas, JE: *Idiopathic orthostatic hypotension: Clinical spectrum and prognosis.* Cardiology 61[Suppl I]:149, 1976.

22. Thomas, JE, et al: *Orthostatic hypotension.* Mayo Clin Proc 56:117–125, 1981.

23. Bannister, R: *Clinical features of progressive autonomic failure.* In Bannister, R (ed): *Autonomic Failure.* Oxford University Press, Oxford, 1983, pp 67–95.

24. Khurana, RK, et al: *Shy-Drager syndrome: Diagnosis and treatment of cholinergic dysfunction.* Neurology 30:805–809, 1980.

25. Evans, DJ, et al: *Idiopathic orthostatic hypotension: Report of an autopsy case with histochemical and ultrastructural studies of the neuronal inclusions.* J Neurol Sci 17:209–218, 1972.

26. Rosen, J and Brown, SI: *New ocular signs in Shy-Drager syndrome.* Am J Ophthalmol 78:1032–1033, 1974.

27. Guilleminault, C, et al: *The impact of autonomic nervous system dysfunction on breathing during sleep.* Sleep 4:263–278, 1981.

28. Lehrman, KL, et al: *Sleep apnea syndrome in a patient with Shy-Drager syndrome.* Arch Intern Med 138:206–209, 1978.

29. Chokroverty, F, Sharp, JT, and Barron, KD: *Periodic respiration and erect posture in Shy-Drager syndrome.* J Neurol Neurosurg Psychiatry 41:980–986, 1978.

30. Chokroverty, S, et al: *The syndrome of primary orthostatic hypotension.* Brain 92:743–768, 1969.

31. Lockwood, AH: *The Shy-Drager syndrome with abnormal respiration and antidiuretic hormone release.* Arch Neurol 33:292–295, 1976.

32. Bannister, R, et al: *Laryngeal abductor paralysis in multiple sytstem atrophy.* Brain 104:351–386, 1981.

33. Hanson, DG, Ludlow, CL, and Bassick, CJ: *Vocal fold paresis in Shy-Drager syndrome.* Ann Otol Rhinol Laryngol 92:85–90, 1983.

34. Thomas, JE and Schirger, A: *Idiopathic orthostatic hypotension: A study of its natural history in 57 neurologically affected persons.* Arch Neurol 22:289–293, 1970.

35. Johnson, RH, et al: *Autonomic failure with orthostatic hypotension due to intermedialateral column degeneration.* Q J Med 35:276–292, 1966.

36. Bannister, R and Oppenheimer, DR: *Degenerative disease of the nervous system associated with autonomic failure.* Brain 95:457–475, 1972.

37. Schwarz, GA: *The orthostatic hypotension syndrome of Shy-Drager.* Arch Neurol 16:123–139, 1967.

38. Oppenheimer, D: *Neuropathology of progressive autonomic failure.* In Bannister, R (ed): *Autonomic Failure.* Oxford University Press, Oxford, 1983, pp 267–283.

39. Sung, JH, Mastri, DR, and Segal, E: *Pathology of Shy-Drager syndrome.* J Neuropathol Exp Neurol 38:353–368, 1979.

40. *Case records of the Massachusetts General Hospital.* N Engl J Med 308:1406–1414, 1983.

41. Lewis, P: *Familial orthostatic hypotension.* Brain 87:719–728, 1964.

42. Bannister, R, Mowbray, J, and Sidgwick, A: *Genetic control of progressive autonomic failure: Evidence for an association with an HLA antigen.* Lancet 1:1017, 1983.

43. Schellong, FS (cited by Luft, R and vonEuler, US): *Two cases of postural hypotension showing deficiency in release of norepinephrine and epinephrine.* J Clin Invest 32:1065–1069, 1953.

44. Demanet, JC: *Usefulness of noradrenaline and tyramine infusion tests in the diagnosis of orthostatic hypotension.* Cardiology 61[Suppl I]:213–224, 1976.

45. Thulesius, O: *Pathophysiological classification and diagnosis of orthostatic hypotension.* Cardiology 61[Suppl I]:180–190, 1976.

46. Polinsky, RJ, et al: *Pharmacological distinction of different orthostatic hypotension syndromes.* Neurology (NY) 31:1–7, 1981.

47. Cryer, PE: *Disorders of sympathetic neural function in human diabetes mellitus: Hypoadrenergic and hyperadrenergic postural hypotension.* Metabolism 29:1186–1189, 1980.

48. Santos, AD, et al: *Orthostatic hypotension: A commonly unrecognized cause of symptoms in mitral valve prolapse.* Am J Med 71:746–750, 1981.

49. Pasternac, A, et al: *Increased plasma catecholamine levels in patients with symptomatic mitral valve prolapse.* Am J Med 73:783–790, 1982.

50. Gaffney, FA, et al: *Autonomic dysfunction in women with mitral valve prolapse syndrome.* Circulation 59:894–901, 1979.

51. Wooley, CF: *Where are the diseases of yesteryear?* Circulation 53:749–751, 1976.

52. Gaffney, AF, et al: *Abnormal cardiovascular regulation in the mitral valve prolapse syndrome.* Am J Cardiol 52:316–320, 1983.

53. Boudoulas, H, et al: *Metabolic studies in mitral valve prolapse syndrome.* Circulation 61:1200–1205, 1980.

54. Coghlan, CH, et al: *Dysautonomia in mitral valve prolapse.* Am J Med 67:236–244, 1979.

55. Leichtman, D, Nelson, R, and Gobel, FL: *Bradycardia with mitral valve prolapse: A potential mechanism of sudden death.* Ann Intern Med 85:453–458, 1976.

56. Streetin, DHP, et al: *Hyperbradykininism: A new orthostatic syndrome.* Lancet 2:1048–1053, 1972.

57. Mathias, CJ and Frankel, HL: *Autonomic failure in tetraplegia.* In Bannister, R (ed): *Autonomic Failure.* Oxford University Press, Oxford, 1983, pp 453–488.

58. Hilsted, J: *Pathophysiology in diabetic autonomic neuropathy.* NY State J Med 82:892–902, 1982.

59. MacKay, JD, Hayakawa, H, and Watkins, PJ: *Cardiovascular effects of insulin: Plasma volume changes in diabetes.* Diabetologia 15:453–457, 1978.

60. Polinsky, RJ, et al: *Pancreatic polypeptide responses to hypoglycemia in chronic autonomic failure.* J Clin Endocrinol Metab 54:48–52, 1982.

61. McGrath, BP, et al: *Impaired pancreatic polypeptide released to insulin hypoglycemia in chronic autonomic failure with postural hypotension: Evidence for parasympathetic dysfunction.* Clin Sci 63:321–323, 1982.

62. Moorhouse, JA, Carter, SA, and Doupe, J: *Vascular responses in diabetic peripheral neuropathy.* Br Med J 1:883–888, 1966.

63. Appenzeller, O and Richardson, ET: *The sympathetic chain in patients with diabetic and alcoholic polyneuropathy.* Neurology (NY) 16:1206–1209, 1966.

64. Cryer, PE: *Normal and abnormal sympathoadrenal function.* NY State J Med 82: 886–891, 1982.

65. Ewing, DJ, et al: *Immediate heart-rate response to standing: Simple test for autonomic neuropathy in diabetes.* Br Med J 1:145–150, 1978.

66. Ewing, DJ, Campbell, IW, and Clarke, BF: *Assessment of cardiovascular effects in diabetic autonomic neuropathy and prognostic implications.* Ann Intern Med 92[Part 2]:308–311, 1980.

67. Leveston, SA, Shak, SD, and Cryer, PE: *Cholinergic stimulation of norepinephrine release in man: Evidence of a sympathetic*

postganglionic axonal lesion in diabetic adrenergic neuropathy. J Clin Invest 64:374–380, 1979.

68. Schenker, VJ, et al: *The effects of ethanol on amine metabolism and alcoholism.* In Maickel, P (ed): *Biochemical factors in alcoholism.* Pergamon Press, Oxford, 1967, p 39.

69. Kyle, RA, Kottke, BA, and Schirger, A: *Orthostatic hypotension as a clue to primary systemic amyloidosis.* Circulation 34:883–888, 1966.

70. Kelly, JJ, Jr, et al: *The natural history of peripheral neuropathy in primary systemic amyloidosis.* Ann Neurol 6:1–7, 1979.

71. Schirger, A, et al: *Orthostatic hypotension in association with acute exacerbations of porphyria.* Proc Staff Meet Mayo Clin 37:7–11, 1962.

72. Siemson, JK and Meister, L: *Bronchogenic carcinoma associated with severe orthostatic hypotension.* Ann Intern Med 58:669–676, 1963.

73. Hennessey, WJ and Siemson, AW: *Autonomic neuropathy in chronic renal failure.* Clin Res 16:385, 1968.

74. Ewing, DJ and Willney, R: *Autonomic function in patients with chronic renal failure on intermittent hemodialysis.* Nephron 15:424–429, 1975.

75. Lilley, JJ, Golden, J, and Stone, RA: *Adrenergic regulation of blood pressure and chronic renal failure.* J Clin Invest 57:1190–1200, 1976.

76. Nies, AS, Robertson, D, and Stone, WJ: *Hemodialysis hypotension is not the result of uremic peripheral autonomic neuropathy.* J Lab Clin Med 94:395-402, 1972.

77. Kalbfleisch, JM and Woods, AH: *Orthostatic hypotension associated with pernicious anemia.* JAMA 1982:196–200, 1962.

78. White, WB, Reik, L, Jr, and Cutlip, DE: *Pernicious anemia seen initially as orthostatic hypotension.* Arch Intern Med 141:1543–1544, 1981.

79. Eisenhofer, G, et al: *Deficient catecholamine release as the basis of orthostatic hypotension in pernicious anemia.* J Neurol Neurosurg Psychiatry 45:1053–1055, 1982.

80. Edmonds, ME, et al: *Autonomic neuropathy in rheumatoid arthritis.* Br Med J 2:173–175, 1979.

81. Carmichael, SM, et al: *Orthostatic hypotension during vincristine therapy.* Arch Intern Med 126:290–293, 1970.

82. McLeod, JG: *Distal autonomic neuropathy.* In Bannister, R (ed): *Autonomic Failure.* Oxford University Press, Oxford, 1983, pp 543–573.

83. Banowitz, NL, et al: *Dihydroergotamine treatment for orthostatic hypotension from vacor rodenticide.* Ann Intern Med 92:387–388, 1970.

84. Long, RG: *Chagas' disease.* In Bannister, R (ed): *Autonomic Failure.* Oxford University Press, Oxford, 1983, pp 596–614.

85. MacLean, AR and Horton, BT: *Myasthenia gravis with postural hypotension.* Proc Staff Meet Mayo Clin 1937, pp 787–792.

86. Schatz, IJ: Unpublished observations.

87. Goldberg, MR, et al: *Selective congenital defect in norepinephrine release as a cause of orthostatic hypotension.* Clin Res 32:332A, 1984.

CHAPTER 4
NEUROGENIC ORTHOSTATIC HYPOTENSION: PATHOPHYSIOLOGIC AND PHARMACOLOGIC INVESTIGATIONS

STUDIES OF PLASMA CATECHOLAMINES

INFUSION OF PRESSOR AGENTS

POSTSYNAPTIC ADRENERGIC RECEPTORS

ANTIDIURETIC HORMONE (ARGININE VASOPRESSIN)

ENZYME MEASUREMENTS

STUDIES OF OTHER PRESSOR AGENTS

In 1948, von Euler[1] showed that norepinephrine (NE) was present in sympathetic nerves; Peart[2] then discovered that it was released when these nerves were stimulated. Current data indicate that NE is stored as granules in sympathetic nerve terminals (Fig. 4-1), where it is protected from monoamine oxidase–induced metabolic degradation.[3] With sympathetic stimulation, the granules are extruded (exocytosis). A complex series of events follows: release of NE into the interstitial space and circulation, but also NE binding to the adrenergic receptor, resulting in receptor stimulation. Norepinephrine is then removed from the synaptic cleft by two mechanisms: reabsorption as granules into the neuron, and

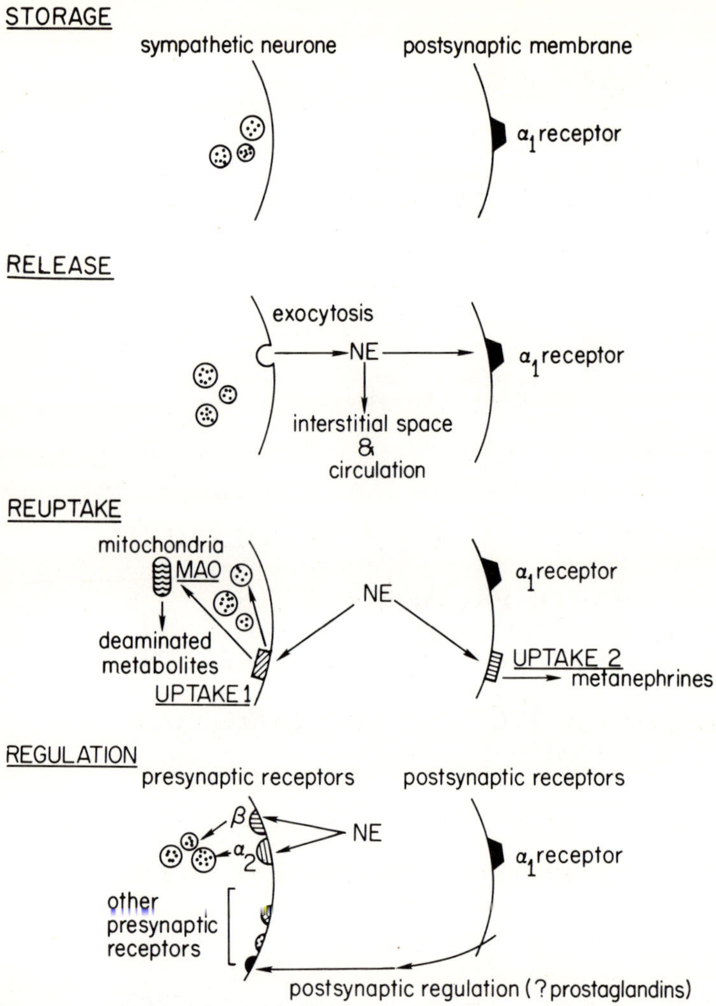

FIGURE 4-1 Schematic representation of regulation of norepinephrine (NE) at nerve terminals.

by metabolism to metanephrine extraneuronally. This entire process has been described as a high-capacity, low-affinity system, ideally suited for removal of catecholamines from the circulation.[4]

Release of NE from neurons is controlled by a complex series of countervailing influences; these include both alpha$_2$ and beta presynaptic receptors, postsynaptic alpha$_1$ receptors, and prostaglandin synthesis and release from postsynaptic sites[5] (see Fig. 4-1).

Knowledge of these facts, plus the development and refinement of sophisticated radioenzymatic techniques to measure plasma catecholamines, has permitted detailed study of sympathetic function in orthostatic hypotension syndromes.

STUDIES OF PLASMA CATECHOLAMINES

As described above, the concentration of NE in the plasma is determined by its release into the circulation from sympathetic neurons after stimulation, and its subsequent removal by reuptake. Measurement of plasma levels during various physiologic and pathologic states could provide important information about normal and abnormal sympathetic function. Meticulous attention, however, must be paid to proper collection, storage, and processing of samples, since a number of perturbing factors may contribute to error.[6] These include the method of venipuncture, and whether the sample is arterial or venous. Nevertheless, knowledge of plasma NE in adequate numbers of patients with orthostatic hypotension, compared with control groups, has provided compelling insights into pathophysiologic mechanisms in these syndromes of orthostatic hypotension.

Such studies indicate that patients with multiple-system atrophy have normal or slightly increased levels of basal NE, but that patients with idiopathic orthostatic hypotension have markedly reduced levels. This clearly implies that there is a different sympathetic defect in multiple-system atrophy when compared with idiopathic orthostatic hypotension[6] (Table 4-1).

Variability within the groups exists, however, and may depend in great part upon the clearance of NE; this would affect the steady-state plasma concentration. Although Esler and colleagues[7] feel that there is delayed clearance of NE in patients with idiopathic orthostatic hypotension, their mea-

TABLE 4-1 Basal Plasma Catecholamines (pg/ml) in MSA* and IOH† (numbers of subjects in parentheses)

Reference	MSA*	IOH†	Controls	Comments
Ziegler et al[22]	310 (6)	95 (4)	315 (10)	Seven patients taking fludrocortisone
Bannister et al[23]	76 (10)	—	550 (4)	One patient had autonomic failure with Parkinson's disease
Bannister et al[24]	214 (8)	30;240 (2)	303;450 (2)	Individual values shown for IOH and controls since only two of each
Esler et al[7]	—	195 (4)	240 (10)	No significant difference between IOH and controls
Polinsky et al[25]	318 (7)	62 (6)	233 (11)	MSA significantly higher and IOH lower than controls. Multiple determinations on each subject
Polinsky et al[26]	255 (7)	91 (5)	—	Predrug assessment for indomethacin trial. No controls

*Multiple-system atrophy
†Idiopathic orthostatic hypotension
Modified from Polinsky,[6] with permission.

surements indicate normal basal plasma NE concentrations. Defective neuronal uptake may explain these findings in this group. An obvious therapeutic implication exists for those patients with delayed removal of NE when given an agent that has indirect sympathomimetic effect.

INFUSION OF PRESSOR AGENTS

It is clear that sensitivity to sympathomimetic agents is altered when sympathetic nerves are damaged.[8] In 1939, Cannon stated that "when in a series of efferent neurons a unit is destroyed, an increased irritability to chemical agents develops in the isolated structure, the effect being maximal in the part being denervated."[9] Thus, direct-acting drugs may produce a more powerful response in denervated subjects, but when complete denervation is present there should be no effect from indirect-acting sympathomimetic agents such as tyramine.

The response of blood pressure (BP) to the infusion of various sympathomimetic agents provides clues to the pathophysiologic process in some syndromes of orthostatic hypotension. Under normal circumstances, the action of tyramine in stimulating peripheral sympathetic nerves requires an intact reuptake mechanism and adequate quantities of NE in nerve endings. The infusion of tyramine in patients with multiple-system atrophy results in a normal or slightly exaggerated vasoconstrictor response. This would suggest that the peripheral (postganglionic) sympathetic system is intact and that the lesion in multiple-system atrophy is presynaptic in location. Conversely, some, but not all, patients with idiopathic orthostatic hypotension have no response to tyramine infusion, whereas others may be supersensitive to it.[6] Clearly, those patients with idiopathic orthostatic hypotension who have no response to tyramine should have complete distal sympathetic neuronal degeneration. Supporting this concept are the findings of an absence of fluorescent staining of catecholamines in blood vessel walls and of reduced catecholamine stores in the skeletal muscle of such patients.[10]

They also should be excessively sensitive to the direct action of exogenous NE, thereby obeying Cannon's law of denervation. Polinsky[6] confirmed this finding in a group of patients with idiopathic orthostatic hypotension (Table 4-2).

Some patients with idiopathic orthostatic hypotension, however, have a supersensitive response to tyramine infusion;[6] the conclusion is inescapable that in this group some nerve endings are still relatively intact and provide a source of NE.

Studies of the action of parenteral NE would directly test the sensitivity of vascular alpha-adrenergic receptors. In normal subjects, NE infusion causes an increase in plasma levels in direct proportion to the rate of administration, and a consequent increase in BP. Patients with multiple-system atrophy demonstrate a somewhat exaggerated response of

TABLE 4-2. Measurement of Plasma Norepinephrine (NE) and Response to Exogenous Catecholamines in IOH and MSA

	Idiopathic orthostatic hypotension (IOH)	Multiple-system atrophy (MSA)
Plasma NE with patient recumbent	Very low	Normal—indicating intact peripheral NE stores
Plasma NE when patient stands	No increase—indicates an inability to stimulate the release of NE	Less than normal response—indicates inadequate stimulus for NE release
Plasma NE response to tyramine infusion	With complete denervation, no response	Normal response—indicates peripheral sympathetic NE stores are available for stimulation
NE infusion	Very marked increase in blood pressure—indicates excessive sensitivity of postganglionic neurons	Normal or slightly exaggerated blood pressure response

mean BP to NE infusion, but those with idiopathic orthostatic hypotension show a very marked hypertensive response, again suggesting supersensitivity of distal sympathetics.

In a series of elegant investigations, Kontos, Richardson, and Norvell[10] studied vascular responses to infused pressors; NE caused a decrease in forearm blood flow in patients with idiopathic orthostatic hypotension, but there was no response to tyramine. Patients with multiple-system atrophy responded normally both to tyramine (diminished flow) and to NE.[10]

Thus, these accumulated data confirm that the lesion in multiple-system atrophy is presynaptic and in idiopathic orthostatic hypotension is postsynaptic (see Table 4-2).

POSTSYNAPTIC ADRENERGIC RECEPTORS

The numbers, binding sites, and degree of affinity of both alpha and beta receptors probably are regulated in great part by the quantities of agonist to which they are exposed.[11] Accordingly, patients with multiple-system atrophy with denervation supersensitivity to infused NE have platelets with elevated levels of alpha receptors.[11] Similarly, increased numbers of lymphocyte beta receptors were measured in a group of patients with multiple-system atrophy, although conflicting data about affinity were observed.[12]

ANTIDIURETIC HORMONE (ARGININE VASOPRESSIN)

"Stretch" or low-pressure receptors in the chest respond to standing by stimulating the release of hypophyseal arginine vasopressin (AVP). The lesions in the brain stem and hypothalamus of patients with multiple-system atrophy interfere with the dopamine and opiate pathways necessary for this AVP feedback loop. Puritz and colleagues[13] demonstrated that the postural stimulation of AVP release was blunted in patients with multiple-system atrophy and that this was due to a loss of dopaminergic and opioid pathways in the brain.

Another study showed an exaggerated pressor response to AVP in patients with multiple-system atrophy.[14] In control subjects, the vasopressor effect of vasopressin is markedly buffered by intrinsically activated cardiovascular reflexes (principally the baroreflex), which would be diminished or absent in patients with multiple-system atrophy.

ENZYME MEASUREMENTS

Black and Petito[15,16] demonstrated normal levels of presynaptic choline acetyltransferase but decreased postsynaptic dopamine-beta-hydroxylase in four patients with idiopathic orthostatic hypotension. They also showed that tyrosine hydroxylase, an enzyme confined to neurons that synthesize dopamine or norepinephrine, was normal in the sympathetic ganglia, but undetectable in the central noradrenergic neurons of the locus ceruleus. Clearly, the primary pathologic process in these patients likely affected both the presynaptic and postsynaptic neurons. Further studies of this kind are needed; in particular, it is essential that the clinical characteristics of the patients studied be documented carefully. Perhaps one or more of the patients described by Black and Petito may have had other neurologic defects in addition to idiopathic orthostatic hypotension.

STUDIES OF OTHER PRESSOR AGENTS

The BP response to the infusion of dopamine was studied in five patients with multiple-system atrophy, five patients with idiopathic parkinsonism, and seven control subjects.[17] A supersensitive response was observed, probably because dopamine has both direct and indirect effects on sympathetic neurons; some evidence exists that denervation causes an increased sensitivity to dopamine.[17,18] Similar studies showed an exaggerated response to methoxamine (a selective alpha agonist) and isoproterenol (a pure beta agonist).[19]

Mathias, Matthews, and Spalding[20] measured renin release during infusion of isoproterenol in a patient with multiple-system atrophy. Profound hypotension and an increase in heart rate occurred, perhaps the result of stimulation of beta-adrenergic receptors in the skeletal muscle, with consequent vasodilatation. The tachycardia could have been related directly to cardiac beta-receptor stimulation, or possibly to vagal withdrawal in response to the hypotension. Basal plasma renin level was normal, and deficient baroreceptor modulation of pressor responses was felt to be the reason for the exaggerated BP response.

Polinsky and coworkers[21] investigated the adrenal medullary reaction to insulin-induced hypoglycemia in eight patients with idiopathic orthostatic hypotension and eight patients with multiple-system atrophy. Plasma glucose, NE, and epinephrine levels were measured; deficient epinephrine responses during insulin tolerance tests were observed. Precise localization of the lesion responsible for the abnormal findings was impossible; dysfunction may have been due to disruption of a number of interrelated factors determining glucose receptor activation and catecholamine release.

REFERENCES

1. Von Euler, US: *Identification of the sympathomimetic ergone in adrenergic nerves of cattle (Sympathin N) with laevo-noradrenaline.* Acta Physiol Scand 16:63–74, 1948.
2. Peart, WS: *The nature of splenic sympathin.* J Physiol (Lond) 108:491–501, 1949.
3. Sever, SA: *Plasma noradrenalin in autonomic failure.* In Bannister, R (ed): *Autonomic Failure.* Oxford University Press, Oxford, 1983, pp 155–173.
4. Iverson, LL: *Role of transmitter uptake mechanisms in synaptic neurotransmission.* Br J Pharmacol 41:571–591, 1971.
5. Langer, SZ: *Presynaptic receptors and the regulation of transmitter release in the peripheral and central nervous system: Phys-*

iological and pharmacological significance. In Usdin, E, Kopin, IJ, and Barchas, J (eds): *Catecholamines: Basic and Clinical Frontiers,* Vol 1. Pergamon Press, New York, 1979, p 387.

6. Polinsky, R: *Pharmacological responses and biochemical changes in progressive autonomic failure.* In Bannister, R (ed): *Autonomic Failure.* Oxford University Press, Oxford, 1983, pp 201–236.
7. Esler, M, et al: *Norepinephrine kinetics in patients with idiopathic autonomic insufficiency.* Circ Res 46[Suppl I]:47–48, 1980.
8. Trendelenberg, V: *Supersensitivity and subsensitivity to sympathomimetic amines.* Pharmacol Rev 15:225–276, 1963.
9. Cannon, WB: *A law of denervation.* Am J Med Sci 198:737–750, 1939.
10. Kontos, HA, Richardson, DW, and Norvell, JE: *Norepinephrine depletion in idiopathic orthostatic hypotension.* Ann Intern Med 82:336–341, 1975.
11. Davies, B: *Adrenergic receptors in autonomic failure.* In Bannister, R (ed): *Autonomic Failure.* Oxford University Press, Oxford, 1983, p 184.
12. Bannister, R, et al: *Beta receptor numbers and thermodynamics in denervation supersensitivity.* J Physiol 319:369–377, 1981.
13. Puritz, R, et al: *Blood pressure and vasopressin in progressive autonomic failure.* Brain 106:503–511, 1983.
14. Mohring, J, et al: *Greatly enhanced pressor response to antidiuretic hormone in patients with impaired cardiovascular reflexes due to idiopathic orthostatic hypotension.* J Cardiovasc Pharmacol 2:367–376, 1980.
15. Black, IB and Petito, CK: *Transynaptic regulation in idiopathic autonomic insufficiency.* Trans Am Neurol Assoc 102:84–86, 1977.
16. Black, IB and Petito, CK: *Catecholamine enzymes in the degenerative neurological disease, idiopathic orthostatic hypotension.* Science 192:910–912, 1976.
17. Wilcox, CS and Aminoff, MJ: *Blood pressure responses to noradrenaline and dopamine infusions in Parkinson's disease and the Shy-Drager syndrome.* Br J Clin Pharmacol 3:207–214, 1976.
18. Marley, E: *Action of some sympathomimetic amines on the cat's iris, in situ or isolated.* J Physiol (Lond) 162:193–211, 1962.

19. Corder, CN, et al: *Postural hypotension: Adrenergic responsivity and levodopa therapy.* Neurology (Minn) 27:921–927, 1977.

20. Mathias, CJ, Matthews, WB, and Spalding, JMK: *Postural changes in plasma renin activity and responses to vasoactive drugs in a case of Shy-Drager syndrome.* J Neurol Neurosurg Psychiatry 40:138–143, 1977.

21. Polinsky, RJ, et al: *The adrenal medullary response to hypoglycemia in patients with orthostatic hypotension.* J Clin Endocrinol Metab 51:1401–1406, 1980.

22. Ziegler, MG, Lake, CR, and Kopin, IJ: *The sympathetic nervous system defect in primary orthostatic hypotension.* New Engl J Med 296:293–297, 1977.

23. Bannister, R, Sever, P, and Gross, M: *Cardiovascular reflexes and biochemical responses in progressive autonomic failure.* Brain 100:327–344, 1977.

24. Bannister, R, et al: *Defective cardiovascular reflexes and supersensitivity to sympathomimetic drugs in autonomic failure.* Brain 102:163–176, 1979.

25. Polinsky, RJ, et al: *Pharmacologic distinction of different orthostatic hypotension syndromes.* Neurology 31:1–7, 1981.

26. Polinsky, RJ, et al: *Effect of indomethacin inhibition of prostaglandin synthesis on blood pressure and plasma norepinephrine levels in patients with orthostatic hypotension.* Neurology 31:63, 1981.

CHAPTER 5

CLINICAL DIAGNOSIS

SYMPTOMS OF INADEQUATE ARTERIAL PERFUSION

SYMPTOMS OF AUTONOMIC DYSFUNCTION

CLINICAL DIAGNOSIS IN THE PATIENT WITH ORTHOSTATIC HYPOTENSION

PHYSICAL EXAMINATION

LABORATORY INVESTIGATIONS

TESTS OF AUTONOMIC FUNCTION

- Valsalva Maneuver
- Modified Noninvasive Valsalva Maneuver

TESTS OF AFFERENT FUNCTION

- Heart Rate Response to Standing
- Amyl Nitrate Inhalation
- Phenylephrine Hydrochloride Injection
- Vasopressin Response to Standing

TESTS OF CENTRAL FUNCTION

TESTS OF EFFERENT FUNCTION

Noninvasive Tests

COLD PRESSOR TEST
ARITHMETIC UNDER STRESS
SWEAT TESTS
EPINEPHRINE INSTILLATION INTO THE EYE
PLASMA NOREPINEPHRINE LEVELS

Invasive Tests

TYRAMINE INFUSION
NOREPINEPHRINE INFUSION

THE CLINICAL USE OF AUTONOMIC FUNCTION TESTING

The manifestations (Table 5-1) of syndromes in which orthostatic hypotension plays a major or prominent role may be divided conveniently into those due to inadequate arterial perfusion and those secondary to autonomic dysfunction. Most often, presenting symptoms and signs are in one or

TABLE 5-1. Initial Symptoms and Signs of Orthostatic Hypotension Syndromes

A. Due to reduced arterial perfusion upon standing
   1. Lightheadedness, dizziness, syncope
   2. Focal cerebral ischemia
   3. Angina pectoris
   4. Postprandial lightheadedness or fainting

B. Due to autonomic dysfunction
   1. Bladder and anal sphincter disturbances
   2. Impotence
   3. Anhidrosis
   4. Parkinsonism-like syndrome
   5. Diffuse neurologic deficits
   6. Supine hypertension
   7. Nasal stuffiness
   8. Night blindness
   9. Sleep apnea
   10. Hoarseness, with laryngeal abductor paresis

the other category; obviously, some overlapping occurs frequently, however.

SYMPTOMS OF INADEQUATE ARTERIAL PERFUSION

The typical complaints of patients with symptomatic orthostatic hypotension upon standing reflect cerebral hypoxia: dizziness, lightheadedness, and sometimes syncope. These may take several minutes to develop, either because the drop in blood pressure (BP) does not occur immediately upon standing, or because the compensatory increase in cerebral blood flow induced by cerebrovascular autoregulation is temporary and loses effectiveness rapidly. It is important to emphasize that such patients do not have these complaints when recumbent; if there is unequivocal evidence that symptoms do occur when the patient is supine, then orthostatic hypotension may be excluded as a cause. Occasionally, however, those with very severe dysfunction have symptoms when sitting up in bed.

If stenosis of the carotid or vertebral-basilar arterial system is present, then a reduction in perfusion across the narrowed lesion, induced by the orthostatic hypotension, may result in focal ischemia of a circumscribed area of brain; symptoms of transient loss of neurologic function consequently appear. These are, in fact, focal ischemic attacks, brought on by orthostatic hypotension. It is essential, therefore, to question each patient who presents with clear-cut transient ischemia as to whether symptoms occur only upon standing.

In some, cerebral blood flow is maintained even in the face of a marked decline in standing BP. Perfusion of other vital organs, however, may be critically diminished, producing ischemia remote from the brain. Thus, patients may have angina pectoris upon standing because of drop in mean arterial blood pressure and the concomitant presence of significant coronary stenosis.[1] Hines, Houston, and Robertson[1] reported that 11 percent of their series of patients with autonomic dysfunction manifested angina pectoris. They point out, however, that a selection factor may occur, in which those patients with significant coronary obstruction probably die early owing to the profound hemodynamic derangements induced by coincident severe orthostatic hypotension.

Postprandial fainting may be the sole presenting sign of orthostatic hypotension. The release of gastrointestinal hormones in response to food likely causes some sequestration of blood in the splanchnic circulation under normal circumstances. If reflex adjustments to standing are blunted or absent, as occurs in orthostatic hypotension, then such pooling of blood could lead to a temporary reduction in effective circulating volume, and would explain why some patients with postural hypotension develop symptoms only after eating.[2]

SYMPTOMS OF AUTONOMIC DYSFUNCTION

Bladder sphincter malfunction manifested by varying degrees of urinary incontinence often may precede the clinical hemodynamic consequences of orthostatic hypotension. Such patients may first be seen by the urologist; it is not unusual for local management to continue for prolonged periods before there is recognition of a general autonomic disturbance with associated orthostatic hypotension. Rarely, anal incontinence may be the initial presenting complaint.

Impotence may precede symptomatic orthostatic hypotension by months, or even years. The careful clinician will always exclude orthostatic hypotension in those male patients in whom the initial complaint is inability to develop or maintain an erection. Anhidrosis provides other evidence of sympathetic dysfunction; most patients complaining of focal dry skin, however, have other indications of autonomic instability.

Unexpected symptoms of lost sympathetic tone are night blindness and nasal stuffiness. The inability to dilate the pupil to accommodate to the dark may be the most troublesome, and sometimes the principal, complaint. Dilated mucosal veins—leading to an irritating sensation of nasal stuffiness—presumably are also caused by inadequate venoconstrictor tone.[2] A therapeutic test, described by Hines and coworkers,[1] is the instillation of phenylephrine eye drops (2.5 percent diluted fourfold). This should result in marked improvement of both the night blindness and the boggy nasal mucosa.

Various central and peripheral nervous system manifestations may appear well before orthostatic hypotension becomes apparent. This pattern occurs in those in whom postural hypotension is the result of baroreceptor reflex arc defects secondary to neurologic disease. Thus, patients with multiple-system atrophy may have focal neurologic deficits reflecting dysfunction of pyramidal, extrapyramidal, or cerebellar systems—for months or years prior to initial signs of orthostatic hypotension.[3]

Patients with a parkinsonism-like picture on initial examination are notorious in this regard. As was pointed out previously, the distinction among idiopathic parkinsonism, idiopathic orthostatic hypotension, and multiple-system atrophy, all with associated orthostatic hypotension, may be most difficult at first. Usually, the orthostatic hypotension in idiopathic parkinsonism is mild, and the extrapyramidal defects predominate. The fact that orthostatic hypotension is not excessively disabling in the patient who presents with parkinsonism-like features favors the initial diagnosis of idiopathic parkinsonism, but careful follow-up is essential.

Even if this assumption turns out to be incorrect and orthostatic hypotension progresses to become the primary management problem, no time has been lost. Delay in the adequate treatment of orthostatic hypotension in no way imparts a prognosis different from that if the patient had been treated vigorously from the time of first consultation with the clinician. The important point is to carefully monitor and document the neurologic findings; such longitudinal follow-up is essential in separating out the various neurologic syndromes and obtaining a sense of the natural course of the disorder in a particular patient.

Symptoms of respiratory dysfunction may be the initial reason for consultation. Vocal cord paresis, producing hoarseness and what has been described as a typical "breathy" voice, may motivate the patient to consult an otorhinolaryngologist. Such complaints are a striking first sign of multiple-system atrophy in some.[4] Various manifestations of sleep apnea syndrome also may be the presenting clue to multiple-system atrophy; these include frank respiratory arrest or periodic respirations or both,[5] usually first witnessed by a spouse.

Supine hypertension, often asymptomatic but occasionally associated with mild headache, is an accompaniment of some syndromes of orthostatic hypotension. The etiology is obscure; a defect in autonomic control of blood vessels is an obvious probability. Antihypertensive agents themselves (see Chapter 2) may lead to orthostatic hypotension; contrariwise, mineralocorticoid drugs (9-alpha-fludrocortisone), used in the treatment of orthostatic hypotension, induce supine hypertension in some cases.

CLINICAL DIAGNOSIS IN THE PATIENT WITH ORTHOSTATIC HYPOTENSION

Once orthostatic hypotension has been established to be present, a meticulous history is necessary to obtain clues to etiology (Table 5-2). This is not merely an exercise in completeness, for the causes of postural hypotension may be benign and short-lived, or may result from progressively disabling neurologic disease. Distinctions among the various possibilities may often be provided by careful and detailed questioning of the patient. Time spent here can obviate fruitless and expensive laboratory investigations.

What medications has the patient been taking in the past 2 to 3 weeks? The pharmacologic half-life in plasma of many compounds is not necessarily the outer limit by which one should exclude a possible effect. For instance, the hypotensive effects of tranquilizer or antidepressant drugs may sometimes persist for 2 to 3 weeks after ingestion, even

TABLE 5-2. Clinical Diagnosis in the Patient With Orthostatic Hypotension

A. *History*
- —*Any* medications
- —Alcohol intake
- —Symptoms of dehydration
- —Neurologic complaints
- —Possible causes of amyloidosis
- —Previous sympathectomy or gastrectomy

B. *Physical Examination*
- —Demonstrate 25/10 mm Hg BP drop on standing; repeat at different times if necessary
- —Do symptoms occur simultaneously?
- —Tilt-table and intra-arterial BPs not necessary
- —Record orthostatic pulse responses
- —Carefully document the extent of neurologic deficit

though the plasma half-life is negligible at that point. Whether this is due to persistent tissue effects, or whether previously suppressed cardiovascular reflexes are sluggish in some patients and need time to recover, is conjectural.

Particular attention must be paid to the use of antihypertensives, tranquilizers, antidepressants, and diuretics. In fact, any agent that interferes with catecholamine secretion, uptake, or utilization, or that affects circulating blood volume is suspect.

Careful evaluation of the patient's history of alcohol intake is essential; although Wernicke's encephalopathy and alcoholic neuropathy are usually seen in patients with markedly excessive alcohol intake, occasionally "moderate" users of alcohol may develop these syndromes.

Are there any symptoms to suggest dehydration? Relatively acute losses of plasma or blood volume are obvious; but occasional patients, particularly those who are elderly and who migrate to warm climates, may have the insidious development of chronic dehydration because of inadequate fluid intake.

Careful neurologic inventory is essential. As has been indicated, symptoms of neurologic deficit may be present well before orthostatic hypotension develops. Attention must be paid to the presence of bladder dysfunction, impotence, anhidrosis, and extrapyramidal defects. Symptoms of peripheral neuropathy may be occult in patients with chronic illness in whom such complaints are either unrecognized or denied. This is particularly true in patients with diabetes mellitus.

Are there any symptoms to suggest amyloidosis, particularly indications of an unexplained neuropathy?

Is there a history of sympathectomy or gastrectomy? These postoperative conditions are sometimes causes of postural hypotension.

Rarely, patients with pheochromocytoma may present with both supine hypertension and orthostatic hypotension. Are the characteristic symptoms of such a tumor (sudden severe headache, palpitations, changes in skin color, and tremulousness) present?

PHYSICAL EXAMINATION

The diagnosis of orthostatic hypotension is made by the demonstration that, within a maximum of 10 minutes of standing without support, there is a drop of at least 25 mm Hg systolic, and 10 mm Hg diastolic in BP. It is important to note whether these signs occur simultaneously with the appearance of symptoms of cerebral hypoxia. If complaints suggest orthostatic hypotension but initial examination does not confirm it, attempts should be made to measure the BP immediately after the patient arises in the morning or, alternatively, soon after eating. There is variability in autonomic control of peripheral vessels, in the competency of the baroreflex arc, and in the intravascular volume status of the patient. Since each of these influences the BP response to standing, failure to demonstrate a significant drop in BP upon standing on one occasion only is insufficient to exclude the diagnosis, particularly if the patient has symptoms of cerebral hypoxia.

Measurement of intra-arterial BP is of no particular added benefit and is usually unnecessary. An exception to this is in very obese patients, where an arm cuff may provide substantially misleading BP measurements.

Similarly, measuring the BP while the patient is on a tilt-table is unwarranted and may, in fact, be misleading. Borst and his colleagues[6] provide data that the cardiovascular responses to active (standing) and passive (tilt-table) changes in posture are fundamentally different. Standing causes involuntary contraction of skeletal muscles, probably influencing afterload and venous return. Such is not the case with head-up tilt, which therefore may induce a greater decline in BP when upright than usually occurs when the same subject stands. Thus, it may be inappropriate to conclude that *significant* orthostatic hypotension is present clinically, if the only substantiation is provided by tilt-table testing, which does not reflect what may be happening clinically.

Many patients are able to measure their own BPs, or have spouses do so. Such records, accompanied by a chart for the tabulation of simultaneous symptoms, are helpful in assessing the clinical severity of the orthostatic hypotension, and in following the effects of management strategies.

The introduction for clinical use of automated BP and pulse recording machines offers an even greater potential for longitudinal evaluation of patients with orthostatic hypotension. Experience with these computerized devices in orthostatic hypotension syndromes has not been reported as yet, however.

Recording the heart rate response to standing is essential. The normal rise of 5 to 15 beats per minute usually is altered in orthostatic hypotension: In those with functional derangements (see Chapter 2), there is usually a compensatory increase in heart rate (more than 20 to 25 beats per minute) owing to enhanced cardioaccelerator (sympathetic) tone, generated in an attempt to increase cardiac output. In those with central nervous system disorders, however, minimal or no increase in heart rate on standing occurs in most patients. These two distinctive responses are exceptionally useful for the clinician: In the one, the compensatory tachycardia strongly implies intact cardiac sympathetics and therefore that functional or sympathicotonic orthostatic hypotension is present; in the other, the lack of pulse response clearly indicates defective cardiac innervation and a neurologic cause of the orthostatic hypotension.

LABORATORY INVESTIGATIONS

Since the diagnosis of orthostatic hypotension usually is clear-cut and straightforward, extensive testing for purposes of differential diagnosis is usually unnecessary. Clearly, the scope of laboratory study depends on the individual patient and his or her associated symptoms and signs. Nevertheless, baseline studies to document the presence or absence of factors that might add to cerebral hypoxia may be necessary. Similarly, even though postural hypotension clearly may be present, other disorders that may further decrease arterial perfusion or tissue oxygenation need to be detected. Thus, the patient with asymptomatic orthostatic hypotension who then develops anemia may cross the threshold from subclinical to overt orthostatic hypotension. As mentioned above, that individual with significant stenosis of the carotid or vertebral-basilar arterial system may have transformed a previously "benign" orthostatic hypotension into physiologically important episodes of cerebral transient ischemia. The older individual with postural hypotension who develops manifestations of the sick sinus syndrome, with alternating episodes of bradyarrhythmia and paroxysmal supraventricular tachycardia, may also develop significant symptoms.

Thus, baseline studies to document the presence or absence of factors that might add to cerebral hypoxia are clearly necessary. These should include measurements of the hemoglobin and hematocrit, arterial Po_2, and the electrocardiogram or 24-hour ambulatory electrocardiogram, or both, to detect cardiac rhythm disturbances. In those patients who present with orthostatic hypotension and some focal sign of neurologic dysfunction, careful selection of neurologic investigations is mandatory. Because mass lesions in the brain stem or in even higher cerebral areas may initially produce postural changes in BP, computed axial tomography of the brain is necessary to exclude tumors and often provides data about the presence of multiple cerebral infarcts. In those who present with evidence of involvement of multiple systems suggestive of multiple-system atrophy, baseline clinical and laboratory measurements are made to follow the progression of the illness.

It is the patient who presents with orthostatic hypotension alone, without any detectable signs of neurologic involvement, in whom a search for an underlying cause is particularly important. Such testing should include the following: hemoglobin-hematocrit, white blood cell count and differential, examination of the peripheral blood film, blood urea nitrogen, serum creatinine, serum electrolytes, 3- or 5-hour glucose tolerance test, 8:00 AM and 3:00 PM plasma cortisol levels, serologic tests for syphilis, and screen of the urine for porphyrins. If there is any suggestion of a peripheral neuropathy of unknown etiology, then it is appropriate to measure immunoglobulins and strongly consider a gingival or rectal biopsy or both to exclude the diagnosis of amyloidosis. If there are no indications of diseases of the peripheral nerves, however, then the value of a blind rectal biopsy for this purpose is arguable.

The extent of the neurologic investigation in patients in whom orthostatic hypotension alone is the only detectable physical finding may be limited. If the syndrome has an organic neurologic basis, then sooner or later obvious symptoms and signs of neurologic impairment will inevitably appear. Unfortunately, early detection of an asymptomatic neurologic disorder usually makes no difference to the natural course of the illness. Thus, there is no compelling reason to proceed with expensive and sometimes invasive tests of central and peripheral nervous systems; most of the reversible or treatable forms of neurologic disease in which orthostatic hypotension occurs either are obvious or may be detected by routine screening, and do not require extensive initial investigations. Lumbar puncture, electroencephalogram, computed axial tomography of the brain, cerebral arteriography, electromyography including nerve conduction studies, and nerve and skin biopsies may be safely delayed until such time as specific indications exist for their use.

In today's climate of consumer activism and medicolegal tension, however, persistent pressure for "a complete investigation" may be inexorable and impossible to resist. In such situations, some or all of the laboratory tests mentioned above should be done to provide a baseline and to assure the patient that everything that can be done has been done to reach a primary diagnosis.

TESTS OF AUTONOMIC FUNCTION

A variety of investigations are available to detect malfunctions of the autonomic nervous system (Table 5-3). Selection of which tests to perform depends on the complexity of the clinical problem and the extent to which documentation of the pathophysiologic site of the lesion will influence subsequent management. Such knowledge may impart a better understanding of natural course and prognosis but may not make much difference in the choice of therapy. Although precise anatomic localization is not usually possible, the portion of the reflex arc that is impaired may be identified by the prudent use of autonomic function testing, together with knowledge of relevant clinical data.

Valsalva Maneuver

The Valsalva maneuver (Fig. 5-1) accurately detects any disturbance in autonomic function, but does not localize it with any degree of anatomic precision. It does require intra-arterial recording of blood pressure.

The test is performed by having the subject exhale against resistance (usually a closed glottis or, more effectively, a closed valve producing a 40-mm Hg pressure gradient). Four distinct phases in the arterial pressure response occur.

Phase 1: An increase in intrathoracic pressure compresses the aorta, causing an abrupt rise in peripheral resistance. This leads to a transient increase in intrathoracic pressure.

TABLE 5-3. Tests of Autonomic Function in Patients With Orthostatic Hypotension

Procedure	Information obtained	Normal response
Valsalva maneuver	Used to document impairment of autonomic function	See Fig. 5-1
Standing	Tests afferent limb (low-pressure baroreceptor integrity)	Heart rate increases 5–15 beats per minute
Amyl nitrite inhalation	Same as above	Tachycardia
Phenylephrine hydrochloride injection	Tests afferent limb (high-pressure baroreceptor integrity)	Bradycardia
Plasma vasopressin	Tests afferent connections (from baroreceptors to neurohypophysis)	Subnormal levels indicate lesion
Hyperventilation	Tests central integrating structures	Hypotension
Cold pressor test	Tests efferent limb	Rise in systolic blood pressure of at least 15 mm Hg
Arithmetic computations with harrassment	Tests efferent limb	Rise in systolic blood pressure
Sweat test	Tests efferent limb	Diffuse sweating
Atropine	Tests efferent vagal fibers	Increased heart rate
Epinephrine hydrochloride drops into eye	Tests end-organ response	Only minor changes in pupil size
Plasma norepinephrine	Tests extra-adrenal stores and end-organ response	Normal at rest; twofold to fourfold increase on standing
Infusion of tyramine and norepinephrine	See text	See text

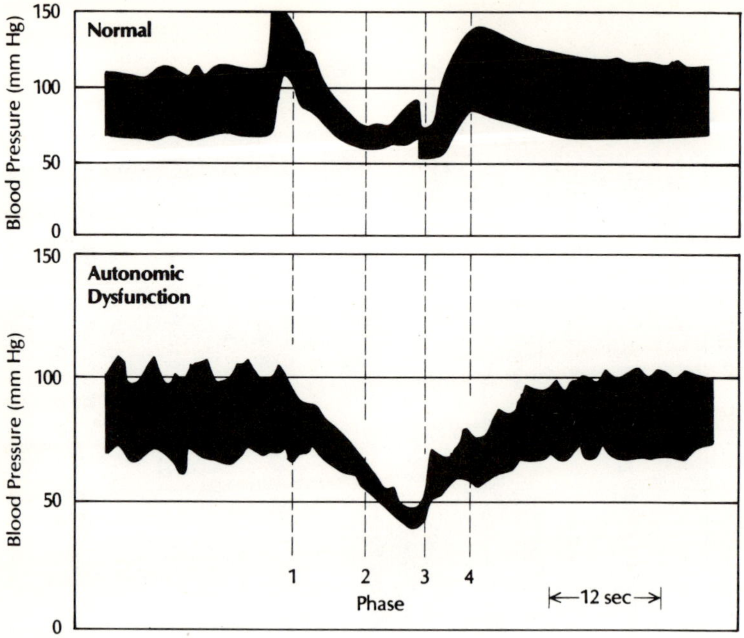

FIGURE 5-1. Valsalva maneuver, with normal response, compared with abnormal response in a patient with idiopathic orthostatic hypotension. After the subject exhales against pressure, an increase in BP normally results (Phase 1), owing to compression of the aorta. During Phase 2, pulse pressure declines because of reduced left ventricular filling; reflex vasoconstriction soon lessens this downward drift. Phase 3 occurs after release of the strain; there is a brief decline in BP. In Phase 4, BP "overshoot" occurs (owing to continuing vasoconstriction), with widened pulse pressure and baroreceptor-mediated bradycardia. In autonomic disorders, defective vasoconstriction and baroreceptors cause a continual downward drift of BP during Phase 2, and neither a BP overshoot nor a bradycardia during Phase 4. (From Schatz, IJ: *Orthostatic hypotension: Diagnosis and treatment.* Hosp Pract 19:67, 1984, with permission.)

Phase 2: This consists of a fall in pulse pressure owing to a decrease in the venous return, left ventricular filling pressure, and cardiac output. The effect varies from subject to subject but is usually reproducible in an individual patient. After 2 to 3 seconds, reflex vasoconstriction causes a plateau in pressure; this is dependent on an intact baroreceptor reflex arc. At the same time, there is a slight increase in heart rate.

Phase 3: A slight drop in mean BP without any change in pulse pressure occurs, and is caused by release of pressure compressing the aorta.

Phase 4: Within 10 seconds of the release of the strain, the systolic and mean BPs rise above the resting level, and the pulse pressure widens. This "overshoot" is caused by the persistent effects of vasoconstriction induced in phase 2; there is usually a return to resting values within 60 seconds after release of the strain. During phase 4, and at the same time as the blood pressure "overshoot" occurs, baroreceptor reflexes initiate a bradycardia to a level below that which occurred in phase 2 and often below the resting level of heart rate.

Reflex vasoconstriction is diminished or absent with autonomic dysfunction; a continual downward drift of the blood pressure during phase 2 results.[7] When the strain is released, the blood pressure "overshoot" and reflex bradycardia do not occur because of inadequate baroreceptor reflexes.

Modified Noninvasive Valvalsa Maneuver

A less accurate reflection of autonomic competence is obtained by using this test noninvasively; the ratio of the maximum heart rate in phase 2 divided by the minimum heart rate in phase 4 is normally greater than 1.25. If less than 1.0 it is considered abnormal, but chronic obstructive lung disease or congestive heart failure may influence the results and render this test unreliable.[7,8]

TESTS OF AFFERENT FUNCTION

Heart Rate Response to Standing

In normal subjects, the heart rate increases anywhere from 5 to 15 beats per minute upon standing; this occurs because diminished baroreceptor stimulation results in an augmented reflex sympathetic discharge to the heart. The usual response of patients with orthostatic hypotension caused by neurologic impairment when upright is a blunting or abolition of this positive chronotropic response to standing. Additionally, there is some inhibition of resting vagal afferent tone.

Patients with orthostatic hypotension secondary to impairment of sympathetic function—at any level of the baroreceptor feedback loop—have little or no increase in heart rate upon standing because of the paralysis of sympathetic drive. On the other hand, patients with orthostatic hypotension in which autonomic function is unimpaired (e.g., volume depletion) or those who have sympathicotonic orthostatic hypotension have a greater than usual increase in heart rate when upright. The compensatory increase in sympathetic tone is an attempt to maintain cardiac output by positive chronotropic and inotropic effects on the heart. Other signs of augmented sympathetic function include pallor and sweating.

It has been suggested that the earliest manifestations of autonomic neuropathy in persons with diabetes are related to initial vagal neuropathy with a consequent increase in resting heart rate.[9] Whether resting tachycardia in diabetic patients without signs of orthostatic hypotension is always due to early vagal neuropathy, creating an imbalance favoring sympathetic cardiac stimulation, or whether there is a relative hypovolemia because of chronic renal protein and salt wasting is conjectural. In any case, these early signs of autonomic neuropathy in persons with diabetes almost always precede by substantial duration the later development of orthostatic hypotension.

Amyl Nitrate Inhalation

Inhalation of amyl nitrate causes marked peripheral vasodilation and a consequent drop in BP. A reflex increase in baroreceptor stimuli to the central nervous system should occur, resulting in compensatory augmentation of sympathetic drive. The most obvious manifestation is tachycardia.

Phenylephrine Hydrochloride Injection

The subcutaneous injection of 50 to 100 micrograms of phenylephrine hydrochloride produces a prompt increase in BP. Diminished baroreceptor impulses to higher centers decrease sympathetic tone, and bradycardia results.

Vasopressin Response to Standing

Vasopressin secretion is stimulated by hypotension and depends on many of the same afferent and central connections responsible for reflex sympathetic activity. Zerbe, Henry, and Robertson[10] measured plasma vasopressin levels lying and upright in 18 patients with orthostatic hypotension. Six had subnormal vasopressin responses when upright, and each had known afferent or central neurologic disease. The remaining 12 patients with orthostatic hypotension had a normal increase in plasma vasopressin; of these, five had peripheral neuropathy, two were dehydrated, and five had unknown disease. Although further corroboration is required, these data suggest that a subnormal response of vasopressin to the upright position indicates a lesion in the central or afferent portion of the reflex arc.

TESTS OF CENTRAL FUNCTION

It is difficult to accurately determine the integrity of the areas in the central nervous system that integrate BP control. With hyperventilation, a fall in the arterial P_{CO_2} causes cerebral vasoconstriction; this, in turn, reduces efferent sympathetic tone abruptly and should result in a decrease in BP. Unfortunately, there is great variability in the response of normal subjects to this test; it is helpful only when there is a drop of at least 20 mm Hg systolic, indicating that central connections are very likely intact.[7]

The vasopressin response to standing (described above)

holds promise as being the most useful measure of central integrity.

TESTS OF EFFERENT FUNCTION

Noninvasive Tests

COLD PRESSOR TEST

The patient's limb is placed in a 4°C ice bath for 60 seconds; normally, there is an increase in systolic BP of at least 15 mm Hg owing to intense reflex vasoconstriction.[11] Confirmation of intact efferent sympathetic innervation may be obtained by plethysmographic monitoring in a contralateral limb; a reflex decrease in flow is demonstrated in a normal subject.

ARITHMETIC UNDER STRESS

A similar increase in systolic BP is demonstrated in patients who perform arithmetic computations under harrassment, presumably owing to augmented catecholamine release and effect. Difficulties arise, however, in quantitating the results of such maneuvers.

SWEAT TESTS

Several methods exist by which sympathetic innervation of sweat glands may be tested. The hand or arm may be placed under a heating lamp or in water at 38°C; rectal temperature should increase by 0.5 to 1.0°C. This increase in body temperature produces sweating if sympathetics are intact.

Another method is to place the patient in a cabinet with a controlled temperature of 46° to 49°C, and a relative humidity of 40 to 50 percent for up to 30 minutes. A powder containing alizarin (a chemical dye that turns purple when moist) is applied to the skin; this should demonstrate diffuse sweating normally. Anhidrosis after the body temperature has risen at least 1°C is an abnormal response.[7] Both methods are cumbersome and little used now.

EPINEPHRINE INSTILLATION INTO THE EYE

If postganglionic sympathetic denervation is present, then hypersensitivity causes the pupil to dilate widely in response to the instillation of one to two drops of 1:1000 epinephrine hydrochloride into the eye. The normally innervated eye demonstrates only minor changes.[12]

PLASMA NOREPINEPHRINE LEVELS

As was discussed in Chapter 4, measurements of plasma norepinephrine (NE) levels in the recumbent position are useful in distinguishing patients with idiopathic orthostatic hypotension from those with multiple-system atrophy or some other central cause of autonomic dysfunction. Patients with idiopathic orthostatic hypotension have extremely low levels (from one-tenth to one-half normal), whereas patients with multiple-system atrophy have normal levels of NE. Studies of patients with amyloid neuropathy and those with diabetes mellitus show that in both groups extremely low levels of recumbent plasma NE also occur.[13,14] This suggests that any neuropathic lesion affecting the postganglionic nerves likely results in marked depletion of plasma NE.

Although measurement of urinary catecholamine levels has been suggested as a substitute, this is usually a cumbersome and imprecise technique for quantifying catecholamine levels.

With standing, there should be no rise in plasma NE levels in either idiopathic orthostatic hypotension or multiple-system atrophy. If some increase in plasma norepinephrine does occur when the patient with idiopathic orthostatic hypotension stands, then it is likely that incomplete denervation is present[15] (see Chapter 4).

Invasive Tests

TYRAMINE INFUSION

Tyramine stimulates the release of stored NE from sympathetic nerve endings. When infused in incremental doses of from 250 μg up to 2000 μg, in normal subjects, this agent induces a systolic BP rise of 25 mm Hg. In patients with idiopathic orthostatic hypotension, there is no response to tyramine because of profound depletion of NE. If a pressure rise is observed, then incomplete postganglionic denervation probably exists. Patients with multiple-system atrophy have a normal response to tyramine.[15]

NOREPINEPHRINE INFUSION

Under normal circumstances, plasma levels of norepinephrine and arterial BP usually increase in direct proportion to the rate of infusion of NE. The usual dose is a mixture of 5 μg of base per 1 ml in 5 percent dextrose in water, given initially at a rate of 2.5 μg per minute. At 10-minute intervals, the infusion rate may be increased to 5, 10, 15, and then 20 μg per minute. The test should be terminated when the systolic BP increases by 40 mm Hg, the diastolic BP increases by 30 mm Hg, the pulse decreases by 30 beats per minute, or any untoward side effects are reported by the patient.[15]

In patients with multiple-system atrophy, there is a somewhat increased BP response to NE when compared with control subjects. Patients with idiopathic orthostatic hypotension, however, have a dramatically exaggerated response of BP to NE infusion when compared with controls.[15] Clearly, extreme caution is necessary when performing these studies in patients with signs of neurologic disease suggestive of idiopathic orthostatic hypotension or multiple-system atrophy.

THE CLINICAL USE OF AUTONOMIC FUNCTION TESTING

These tests are useful only insofar as they may provide a better understanding of prognosis and help make management more effective. Obviously, careful selection of those studies that provide the most information at the least risk is mandatory. If the clinical data give an obvious clue to the anatomic site of the pathophysiologic lesion, then a minimum of testing is necessary. The noninvasive tests are generally time consuming and not very precise, and each of the invasive tests has some hazard.

The Valsalva maneuver indicates that there is a defect somewhere in the reflex arc but does not localize it. Investigations of efferent sympathetic function, principally the cold pressor test, provide important information as to the integrity of that part of the reflex loop. If, however, the result of the Valsalva maneuver is abnormal, and that of the cold pressor test is normal, then the inference is clear that the lesion is either central or in the afferent limb. If, on the other hand, the cold pressor test indicates efferent dysfunction, then measurement of plasma NE with the patient recumbent often provides important data about whether the disorder is preganglionic or postganglionic, and thus distinguishes multiple-system atrophy from idiopathic orthostatic hypotension (or some other peripheral lesion).

It is rarely necessary to employ more extensive investigations of sympathetic function such as the infusion of tyramine, norepinephrine, or angiotensin II. These studies probably are best done in research centers and are used principally for the elucidation of basic pathophysiologic mechanisms.

On balance, the routine use of the cold pressor test and basal plasma NE levels provides important information at low cost and no risk. Even these may not be necessary in the patient who presents with clear-cut signs of a primary neurologic lesion in whom orthostatic hypotension is a secondary phenomenon, or where the clinical situation clearly indicates multiple-system atrophy. It is in those patients with orthostatic hypotension as the principal sign with minimal or no neurologic symptoms that utilization of autonomic function tests may be of some practical benefit to the patient.

REFERENCES

1. Hines, S, Houston, M, and Robertson, D: *The clinical spectrum of autonomic dysfunction.* Am J Med 70:1091–1096, 1981.
2. Robertson, D, Wade, D, and Robertson, RM: *Postprandial alterations in cardiovascular hemodynamics in autonomic dysfunctional states.* Am J Cardiol 48:1048–1052, 1981.
3. Schatz, IJ, Podolsky, S, and Frame, B: *Idiopathic orthostatic hypotension: Diagnosis and treatment.* JAMA 171:537–540, 1963.
4. Bannister, R, et al: *Laryngeal abductor paralysis in multiple system atrophy.* Brain 104:351–386, 1981.
5. Lehrman, KL, et al: *Sleep apnea syndrome in a patient with Shy-Drager syndrome.* Arch Intern Med 138:206–209, 1978.
6. Borst, C, et al: *Mechanisms of initial heart rate response to postural change.* Am J Physiol 243:H676–H681, 1982.
7. Henrich, WL: *Autonomic insufficiency.* Arch Intern Med 142:339–344, 1982.
8. Thomas, JE, et al: *Orthostatic hypotension.* Mayo Clin Proc 56:117–125, 1981.
9. Ewing, DJ, Campbell, IW, and Clark, BF: *Assessment of cardiovascular effects in diabetic autonomic neuropathy and prognostic implications.* Ann Intern Med 92(2):308–311, 1980.
10. Zerbe, RL, Henry, DP, and Robertson, GL: *Vasopressin response to orthostatic hypotension.* Am J Med 74:265–271, 1983.
11. Godden, JO, Roth, GM, and Hines, EA, Jr: *The changes in the intraarterial pressure during emersion of the hand in ice cold water.* Circulation 12:963–973, 1965.

12. Thompson, PD and Melmon, KL: *Clinical assessment of autonomic function.* Anesthesiology 24:724–731, 1968.

13. Suzuki, T, et al: *Orthostatic hypotension in familial amyloid polyneuropathy treatment with DL-threo-3.4-dihydroxyphenylserine.* Neurology 31:1323–1326, 1981.

14. Neubauer, B and Christensen, NJ: *Norepinephrine, epinephrine, and dopamine contents of the cardiovascular system in long term diabetes.* Diabetes 25:6–10, 1976.

15. Polinsky, RJ, et al: *Pharmacologic distinction of different orthostatic hypotension syndromes.* Neurology 31:1–7, 1981.

CHAPTER 6
MANAGEMENT

GENERAL MEASURES

PHYSICAL MEASURES

- Head-Up Tilt at Night
- Lower Body External Pressure

PHARMACOLOGIC MEASURES

- Fludrocortisone Acetate
- Vasopressors
- Ergot Derivatives
- Prostaglandin Inhibition
- Adrenergic Blockers
- Miscellaneous Agents

MECHANICAL DEVICES

The goal of treatment should be to reduce the symptoms of inadequate organ perfusion (Table 6-1). The hypotensive patient without symptoms of cerebral hypoxia usually does not need specific therapy, since cerebral autoregulation may be effective at levels of even 70-mm Hg systolic blood

TABLE 6-1. Management of Orthostatic Hypotension

A. 1. Eliminate or diminish any condition that prevents venous return or decreases left ventricular filling.
   2. When standing, should continuously flex calf muscles.
   3. Eat frequent small meals, and avoid sudden standing after eating.
   4. Arise slowly from bed in the morning.
   5. Avoid straining at stool.

B. Treat specific primary diseases, if possible.

C. Apply physical measures.
   1. Keep head and trunk tilted upward at night.
   2. Wear counterpressure support garment.

D. Pharmacologic therapy (see text).
   1. Fludrocortisone acetate.
   2. Vasopressors (phenylephrine, ephedrine, amphetamine, midodrine [investigational], hydroxyamphetamine, methylphenidate, tyramine, prenalterol).
   3. Ergot derivatives (investigational).
   4. Prostaglandin inhibitors.
   5. Beta-adrenergic blockers
   6. Clonidine.

E. Atrial pacing.

F. Mechanical devices (investigational).

pressure (BP). The one important exception to this occurs in those with coronary artery obstructive disease with orthostatic hypotension; they may develop asymptomatic myocardial ischemia, reflected by significant ST segment changes on ambulatory electrocardiographic recording. In such patients, orthostatic hypotension must be treated vigorously, even in the absence of either cerebral hypoxia or overt angina pectoris.

Although I have focused on disturbances of the baroreflex arc as the usual cause of neurogenic orthostatic hypotension, the long-term adjustment to orthostatic hypotension is probably determined more by the control of blood volume through low-pressure receptors in the kidney, by antidiuretic hormone release, and by the renin–aldosterone–angiotensin mechanism. Recumbent hypertension often develops in these patients either because of defective baroreceptor reflexes or as a consequence of therapy with volume expansion. Theoretically, such hypertension can lead to an increase in cerebral vascular resistance, which in turn enhances cerebral ischemia upon standing.

It is likely of critical importance, therefore, that initial management should enable the patient to become mobile, for even a temporary ability to stand enhances intrinsic homeostatic responses to the upright position. This, in turn, causes an increase in extracellular fluid volume and an improvement in myogenic tone.[1] The hope is that a self-perpetuating phenomenon will begin to operate, in which intrinsic compensatory mechanisms play a favorable role.

Most patients derive substantial benefit from a properly chosen and judiciously monitored treatment program. Nonetheless, the physician should avoid implications that therapy will favorably alter the natural history of the specific disorder that is present; in general, the rate of progression cannot be predicted. This is particularly true in patients with neurogenic orthostatic hypotension, although there are some data to suggest that idiopathic orthostatic hypotension has a more benign course. A mixture of treatment modalities best suited for the individual is usually necessary; this requires an educated and cooperative patient and a reassuring and understanding physician.

GENERAL MEASURES

Any condition that favors the pooling of blood and where venous return is impeded must be eliminated or diminished, if possible. Obviously, specific therapy aimed at a secondary disease process that has caused postural hypotension should be instituted. In addition to this, however, there is some general advice that is given to patients with symptomatic orthostatic hypotension.

1. When the patient is upright or standing, he or she should be instructed to flex the calf muscles and to avoid standing still in one place, in order to enhance the venous pump and therefore increase venous return.

2. Patients often learn to abort disabling symptoms of cerebral hypoxia by squatting; the embarrassment of this maneuver may be diminished or obviated by advising the patient to carry a small collapsible chair.

3. Postprandial hypotension and consequent symptoms are a significant problem for some patients; the simple expedient of eating frequent, smaller meals and avoiding sudden standing may substantially reduce these episodes.

4. Similarly, patients should be instructed not to rise too quickly from a supine position, particularly upon arising in the morning. Symptoms are almost always worse at that time; therefore, this simple precaution may diminish disability.

5. Occasionally, straining at stool mimics the Valsalva maneuver. Patients should be told to avoid this, and they should be given stool softeners, as necessary.

6. Careful attention to the effect of general anesthesia on BP control during operative procedures is essential:

a. Basal BP is determined in great part by the state of hydration and the positioning of the patient.
b. Positive-pressure respiration may induce hypotension, similar to that seen in phase 2 of the Valsalva maneuver.
c. Some anesthetic agents, as well as drugs used in the operative period, may induce marked variability in blood pressure.
d. Midbrain respiratory control may be abnormal.
e. Aberrations of vagal tone alter the effect of atropine.
f. Abnormalities of sweating and pupillary response may interfere with adequate monitoring.
g. The adrenal medulla may not react appropriately to surgical stress.

Clearly, this litany of potential problems makes imperative close liaison among attending physician, surgeon, and anesthesiologist; meticulous monitoring of the patient during and after operation is required.[2,3]

PHYSICAL MEASURES

Head-Up Tilt at Night

The head-up tilt at night maneuver was first proposed by Maclean and Allen[4] in 1940. Clear evidence is now available that blood volume increases by its use.[5] Nocturnal head-up body tilt probably functions by reducing renal arterial pressure and prompting renin release, with consequent angiotensin II formation, aldosterone stimulation, and an increase in blood volume; obviously, this is true only in those patients who can still release renin.[6] Fortunately, most patients with neurogenic orthostatic hypotension maintain this capability.

Lower Body External Pressure

Applying graduated pressure to the lower half of the body (Fig. 6-1) substantially reduces venous pooling when upright and thus increases central blood volume, left ventricular filling pressure, cardiac output, and cerebral perfusion. This is best accomplished by the use of a custom-fitted, commercially available counterpressure support garment, made of elastic mesh which forms a single unit extending from the metatarsals to the costal margins.[7] It is so constructed that pressure is maximum at the ankles and less at the waist. Eventually, most patients learn to tolerate the use of this garment, but the initial motivation must be strong, since maximum utility requires that it be worn at all times when upright. In my experience, it is less acceptable to patients in tropical and semitropical climates, even though the material is porous. The benefit that patients obtain from the use of such counterpressure is often impressive and sometimes eliminates the need for pharmacologic treatment of orthostatic hypotension. A theoretical objection that such external pressure reduces the myogenic reaction to stretch, which is present even in partially denervated vessels, is out-

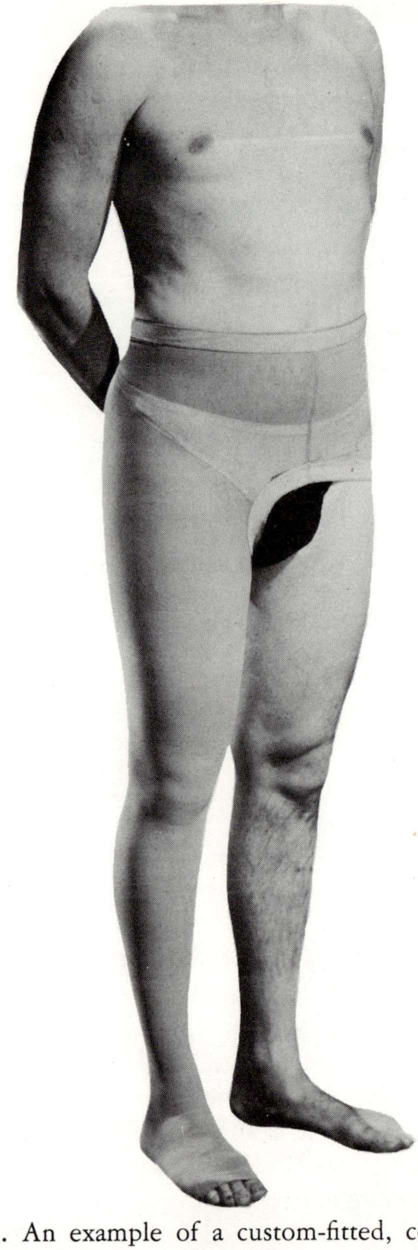

FIGURE 6-1. An example of a custom-fitted, counterpressure support garment, worn from metatarsals to waist. (Photo courtesy of Jobst Institute, Inc., Toledo, OH.).

weighed by the value of increasing central blood volume and left ventricular filling pressure.[8]

In my own experience, physical measures alone (head-up tilt at night and waist-length leotard) sometimes are sufficient therapy in patients with mild symptomatic orthostatic hypotension. Except for those with occult coronary disease, the objective is to *relieve symptoms,* and not merely to regain normal levels of BP. The patient who is dizzy and weak with systolic blood pressures of 70, but is asymptomatic when pressure is 85 after initiating physical measures, is managed successfully. The only caveat is that a 24-hour ambulatory electrocardiogram be obtained to exclude occult myocardial ischemia when standing.

If physical measures are unsuccessful, then attempts at drug therapy are appropriate. Successful pharmacologic treatment, however, is difficult; the balance between sympathetic and parasympathetic stimuli and the exquisitely delicate central integration of many afferent impulses that normally exist are impossible to emulate by the use of exogenous chemicals. The agents available to us cannot be considered adequate replacements for naturally occurring neurotransmitters. Nevertheless, capitalizing on receptor supersensitivity and utilizing a step-by-step approach oftentimes result in a decrease of functional impairment in the patient.

PHARMACOLOGIC MEASURES

Unfortunately, no single agent is uniformly successful. Trials of drugs, sometimes consecutively and sometimes concurrently, are needed in order to identify the best treatment program for an individual patient. Often, a combination of compounds is successful in one patient and not in another, and yet the disease process appears to be the same in both. Thus, considerable manipulation of physical measures and individual drug programs is usually required for each patient; in general, the practitioner who perseveres will find a regimen that is successful in substantially reducing disability from orthostatic hypotension.

Success judged by empirical results from personal experience of treating one or several patients is a realistic yardstick for the physician to use. Most published reports of therapy are anecdotal in nature, lack rigorous controls and crossover designs, and have insufficient numbers of study patients from whom to draw valid scientific conclusions about effectiveness. As a consequence, individual experience may be used as an acceptable substitute to provide therapeutic guidelines (Table 6-2).

Fludrocortisone Acetate

Fludrocortisone acetate (Table 6-3) is the cornerstone of drug therapy in orthostatic hypotension, and I favor its initial use in all patients, unless there is some obvious contraindication. There is a uniform expansion of plasma volume, but this does not persist in all patients permanently. Multiple other pharmacologic effects of fludrocortisone include:

1. Augmenting norepinephrine release from the remaining normal sympathetics and thus increasing effective vasoconstriction on standing.
2. Probably sensitizing vascular receptors to pressor amines in both control subjects and in patients with orthostatic hypotension.[9]

TABLE 6-2. Author's Approach to Management

1. Apply general and physical measures as outlined, with particular emphasis on counterpressure support garment.
2. If pharmacologic therapy is still necessary, institute fludrocortisone.
3. Establish maximum tolerated daily dose and monitor for complications.
4. Add indomethacin, if necessary.
5. If necessary, add pindolol.
6. If significant, symptomatic hypotension is still present, reevaluate and consider ergotamine tartrate or clonidine.

TABLE 6-3 Putative Pharmacologic Effects of Fludrocortisone

1. Expanded plasma volume
2. Augmented norepinephrine release
3. Increased vascular reactivity to norepinephrine
4. Increased fluid content of vascular wall
5. Enhancement of adrenergic receptor sites

3. Increasing the fluid content of the vascular wall and therefore enhancing vasoreactivity.
4. In patients with idiopathic orthostatic hypotension, there are greater numbers of alpha- and beta-receptor sites on lymphocytes than in control patients. These receptor numbers are further enhanced after treatment with fludrocortisone.[10]

As Bannister has pointed out,[1] aldosterone secretion is usually reduced in patients with neurogenic orthostatic hypotension, but the defect is probably the result of chronic reduction of angiotensin stimulation of aldosterone production rather than a primary adrenal defect. Fludrocortisone, therefore, may increase blood volume by becoming a pharmacologic substitute for aldosterone. In order to avoid overloading the circulation, delicate adjustments of dosage are needed for each patient.

The initial dose of fludrocortisone is 0.1 mg daily; this may be increased by increments of 0.1 mg every 5 to 7 days. Maintenance varies from 0.1 to 1.0 mg daily and is limited by the presence of complications from the medication. These include recumbent hypertension, marked fluid retention, frank congestive heart failure, and hypokalemia. In a series of patients treated with fludrocortisone, these complications were present in approximately 30 percent of patients[11] (Table 6-4). Although such a complication rate is high, their appearance is not necessarily an immediate indication for termination of therapy. Each of these conditions may be treated effectively by appropriately targeted therapy. If successful, such treatment will permit continuation of fludrocortisone. Since patients vary in response and in the inci-

TABLE 6-4. Complications of Fludrocortisone

1. Supine hypertension
2. Fluid retention
3. Congestive heart failure
4. Hypokalemia
5. Enhancement of diabetes mellitus

dence of complications, meticulous clinical monitoring is mandatory. Mathias[12] has observed occasional tachyphylaxis, and feels that this problem can be managed by increasing the dose of fludrocortisone, if it is tolerated by the patient.

Occasionally, an evening and morning dosage schedule may provide smoother BP maintenance than a once-daily ingestion of the drug.

The concomitant use of a high sodium intake of at least 150 mEq per day is also advisable, if acceptable to the patient. In fact, self-medication with sea water was used successfully in one patient.[40]

Vasopressors

Vasopressors were the first drugs used in attempts to treat orthostatic hypotension. In general, their effectiveness varied inversely with the extent of the disease; in patients with mild orthostatic hypotension, who probably could have been managed successfully by physical measures and sound general advice, these agents were described as being particularly useful. Unfortunately, the converse was true in those with severe and disabling orthostatic hypotension.

Ephedrine, which acts both directly and indirectly on the sympathetic nervous system, and phenylephrine, which is a direct alpha agonist, have been utilized. Supine hypertension is often a complication of adequate ephedrine therapy, and it also may be addictive, presumably because of its central effect.[1] Theoretically, direct-acting alpha agonists such as phenylephrine and midodrine would be particularly useful in treatment of those with decreased norepinephrine (NE) stores, or reduced plasma levels. However, the same problem of recumbent hypertension was observed in a group of patients treated with phenylephrine; although approximately one third had a beneficial effect from this agent, the presence of high BP when recumbent diminished its usefulness.[13]

Midodrine is an alpha-receptor agonist with consequent constrictor action on both the arterioles and the veins and little or no cardiac positive inotropic or chronotropic activity. Initial reports on the use of this agent are encouraging, although it should be noted that some of the patients receiving the drug required additional therapy (usually beta-adrenergic blocking drugs) to control supine hypertension.[14]

Other pressors that have been recommended, principally by Thomas and coworkers[15] at the Mayo Clinic, include methylphenidate and hydroxyamphetamine. My own experience, however, is that when used alone these agents are usually without any significant effect on orthostatic hypotension; if given in combination with other agents, they sometimes may have an additive effect.

Prenalterol, a selective beta agonist, was reported to be successful in a single case of multiple-system atrophy.[41]

Tyramine, which causes the release and reuptake of NE, may be given orally. Unfortunately, it is degraded in the intestine and therefore has little pharmacologic effect upon absorption. In 1970, Diamond, Murray, and Schmid[16] suggested that the concomitant use of a monoamine-oxidase inhibitor with tyramine would prevent intestinal degradation and thus would permit appropriate action. There was initial enthusiasm for this therapy, but BP responses proved to be erratic. Tyramine was given in the form of cheddar cheese, and sometimes marked hypertension resulted, presumably from an inexact titration of the amount of tyramine in the aliquot of cheese served. Interest has waned because of the unpredictability of BP control. In addition, it is possible that in patients with idiopathic orthostatic hypotension who have some remaining intact postganglionic sympathetics that are able to release NE, supersensitivity may result in very severe hypertension.

Ergot Derivatives

In 1970, it was first demonstrated that dihydroergotamine could elicit a powerful vasoconstrictor action on the veins of the hand.[17] Recent studies by Chobanian and coworkers[18] confirmed these data, and also suggested that the vascular effect was principally due to venoconstriction in both the recumbent and upright positions.

It is likely that these agents produce alpha-adrenergic stimulation, although their action may differ from that of NE.[17,19] The pharmacologic activity may be based upon a serotonin-mediated mechanism, which cannot be affected by phentolamine (an alpha-adrenergic blocker); in part, it also may be mediated through the prostaglandin system.[20,21] The final pharmacologic result is an increase in central blood volume and left ventricular filling pressure.

Dihydroergotamine is highly effective in patients with idiopathic orthostatic hypotension when given parenterally; unfortunately, when administered by mouth, it has a very low bioavailability.[22] This may be due to high first-pass removal by the liver. It has been suggested that combining it with nitroglycerin might increase its absorption from the gut.[23]

Ergotamine tartrate, however, was recently reported to be effective in a limited study in four patients[18] (Table 6-5). There is an obvious difference in effect between these two agents, presumably based upon varying rates of bioavailability. Chronic oral administration in this investigation was successful: marked clinical improvement without significant recumbent hypertension occurred. Platelet alpha-receptor numbers were reduced toward normal (Table 6-6).

A general concern about the use of ergot derivatives would be their known potential for stimulating cerebral and coronary arterial constriction in susceptible subjects. At present, therefore, further rigorous study of the potential for practical use of these agents in treating patients with orthostatic hypotension is necessary before any recommendations are warranted.

TABLE 6-5. Clinical Effects of Ergotamine Bitartrate in Patients with Chronic Orthostatic Hypotension

Pt	Dose (mg/day)	BP (mm Hg) Control period		BP (mm Hg) Treatment period						Syncope/Presyncope (# per week)		Other
				1 Month		3 Month		6 Month				
		Rec	Up	Rec	Up	Rec	Up	Rec	Up	Control	Ergot	
1	2	148 ± 3/85 ± 2	52 ± 4/32 ± 4	164/90	104/60	146/82	96/62	166/88	102/64	3.2	0.2	Marked increase in physical activity with treatment
2	4	128 ± 5/64 ± 4	48 ± 6/28 ± 5	148/82	76/50	—	—	—	—	4.8	2.4	Ergotamine ineffective during periods of anorexia and dehydration
3	3	116 ± 4/60 ± 3	66 ± 7/36 ± 6	90/60	80/50	110/70	90/60	110/80	90/62	7.0	0.5	Marked increase in physical activity with treatment
4	2	72 ± 4/40 ± 2	42 ± 2/24 ± 3	104/68	92/70	94/72	90/66	94/62	90/64	4.0	0	No postural symptoms during ergotamine therapy

Blood pressure values represent the mean ± SEM.
Blood pressure was measured 1–3 hours after administration of ergotamine.
BP = blood pressure; Rec = recumbent; Up = upright.
From Chobanian et al,[18] with permission of the author and the American Heart Association, Inc.

TABLE 6-6. Effects of Ergotamine Therapy on Platelet Alpha-receptor Affinity and Number in Patients with Orthostatic Hypotension

Pt	Plasma norepinephrine (ng/ml)		Pressor responsiveness to infused norepinephrine	Platelet α Receptor			
				K_D (nM)		Number (per platelet)	
	Recumbent	Upright		Control	Ergot*	Control	Ergot*
1	0.098	0.125	Increased	11.7	12.5	345	105
2	0.140	0.184	Increased	10.0	7.2	430	228
3	0.175	0.160	Increased	11.1	7.8	455	264
4	0.285	0.320	Normal	11.5	9.6	332	145

Control subjects (n = 20)
Plasma norepinephrine (recumbent) 0.284 ± 0.20 mg/ml
Plasma norepinephrine (upright) 0.464 ± 0.038 ng/ml
Platelet K_D for [^{3}H] dihydroergocryptine 12.4 ± 1.3 × 10 nM
Platelet α-receptor number 234 ± 17/platelet
*Values represent the average of two separate assays performed between 2 and 6 weeks of ergotamine therapy.
K_D = disappearance rate
From Chobanian et al,[18] with permission of the author and the American Heart Association, Inc.

Prostaglandin Inhibition

The use of an agent that suppresses prostaglandin synthesis, such as indomethacin, was first suggested as a means of preventing vasodilatation in 1978.[24] Improvement was reported in four patients with orthostatic hypotension, but subsequent confirmation of the utility of such agents has not been available. Indomethacin increases sensitivity to infused NE in some patients with neurogenic orthostatic hypotension, but the pressor effect noted was unfortunately only significant on supine BP.[1] It has been speculated, therefore, that prostaglandin inhibition increases the vasoconstrictive capabilities of endogenous NE available from whatever intact nerve endings exist. Other data reported "some" improvement in a group of 12 patients with orthostatic hypotension.[25]

At present, the information available is inadequate to describe with any precision the pharmacologic action on blood vessels. Experience suggests that indomethacin, when used alone, is rarely successful in raising BP significantly. However, the combination of prostaglandin inhibition with fludrocortisone may have an additive effect in increasing smooth-muscle sensitivity to endogenous NE and, in addition, may cause substantial increases in blood volume.[26]

Adrenergic Blockers

In 1966, it was suggested that beta-agonist–induced vasodilatation might contribute to orthostatic hypotension.[27] Propranolol use was predicated on this assumption. Theoretically, beta blockade might further increase the adrenal release of catecholamines; this sometimes occurs after exercise in subjects treated with beta-blocking drugs.[28]

In 1977, Chobanian and coworkers[29] obtained good results by giving propranolol to four patients with neurogenic orthostatic hypotension who were already taking fludrocortisone. Other data are less encouraging, however, and, in general, beta blockade with propranolol has not proved efficacious.

In those patients with the rare syndrome of hyperbradykininism, anecdotal experience suggests that propranolol is most useful, however.

The major indication for the use of beta blockade probably rests with those who have sympathicotonic orthostatic hypotension, in which excessive tachycardia upon standing occurs; propranolol given to these patients is almost uniformly effective in reducing excessive sympathetic discharge. The theoretical use of a combined alpha- and beta-blocking agent, such as labetalol, is attractive since there may be both excessive alpha and beta activity in this group of patients. However no data are published in this area.

Pindolol is much more promising for use in orthostatic hypotension, because it has significant intrinsic sympathomimetic action. The initial speculation about the use of this compound was based on the presumption that when adrenergic receptor occupancy was low, as occurs in the postganglionic lesion of idiopathic orthostatic hypotension, even a partial beta agonist—such as pindolol—would act as a full agonist; furthermore, its action would be greatly enhanced by denervation hypersensitivity and defective baroreflexes.[30] Pindolol might also increase venous tone, probably by action on venous beta receptors. Unfortunately, its initial use resulted in no change in vascular resistance, although an improved cardiac output caused less orthostatic hypotension. Subsequently, Davidson and Smith[31] observed no benefit from the use of pindolol in three patients with autonomic neuropathy and in two with amyloidosis. Other reports also cast some doubt upon the efficacy of this agent because of varying responses.[32]

It is probable that these data are conflicting because insufficient attention was paid to the site of the lesion.[33] It may be that pindolol is most effective in idiopathic orthostatic hypotension, where it likely acts as an almost pure agonist because of the marked degrees of denervation supersensitivity. Man in't Veld, Boomsma, and Schalekamp[33] claim that if a small intravenous dose of pindolol (0.4 to 0.8 mg) produces an increase in heart rate, then this suggests a combination of low receptor occupancy and increased receptor number and/or receptor sensitivity in patients with idiopathic orthostatic hypotension. In those with a preganglionic efferent lesion (patients with multiple-system atrophy), however, no heart rate change would be expected, and therefore the clinical usefulness of pindolol would be diminished or absent. Obviously, further extensive and rigorous clinical pharmacologic testing of pindolol is warranted, but at present its judicious use, particularly in patients with clear-cut idiopathic orthostatic hypotension, would be justified.

Miscellaneous Agents

Clonidine is a partial alpha-receptor agonist with both central and peripheral actions. Recently, it was used in four patients with idiopathic orthostatic hypotension in the dosage of 0.8 mg daily.[34] The results were considered to be generally favorable, although some complications were observed, including excessive recumbent hypertension.

A number of compounds, used either in the treatment of multiple-system atrophy or to counteract the aggravated orthostatic hypotension due to antiparkinsonian drugs, have been suggested. L-dopa creates hypotension that is centrally mediated; it also replenishes stores of peripheral NE, and it may enhance adrenergic transmission in the baroreflex arc. It might, therefore, increase the response of peripheral vessels to standing. Occasional patients are reported to benefit from its use, when its peripheral actions predominate.[1]

Metoclopramide is a drug that inhibits the vasodilator effects of excessive dopamine; it therefore has been used in some patients with orthostatic hypotension.[35] Because central dopamine receptors may be supersensitive in some persons, extrapyramidal side effects may be exaggerated.[1] Other dopamine agonists such as lisuride and pergolide have shown little promise.[1]

The use of atrial tachypacing should be considered in occasional patients who have bradycardia and orthostatic hypotension.[36,44] The resulting increase in cardiac output is due both to a more rapid heart rate and to the positive inotropic effect on ventricular contractility of the tachycardia.[43] Before making a commitment to permanent dual-chamber (atrioventricular sequential) pacing, however, careful measurement of the increase in cardiac output achieved by temporary "physiologic" pacing is mandatory. Such studies need to be performed in the cardiac laboratory, with the patient upright, and intra-arterial blood pressure recorded. Suitable patients, carefully selected and tested, may be helped substantially by this procedure.

In a single case report, the administration of combined H-1 and H-2 receptor antagonists, in a patient with diabetic autonomic failure and orthostatic hypotension, was reported successful.[37] Effectiveness was ascribed to the inhibition of certain in vivo actions of histamine.

Caffeine (250 mg) was found to be useful in improving postprandial hypotension in a placebo-controlled study.[42] Plasma catecholamine levels were not affected significantly; it was concluded, therefore, that caffeine acted as a pressor agent independent of sympathoadrenal function. Whether the use of this agent will result in practical benefits to patients needs further assessment.

MECHANICAL DEVICES

Recently, Polinsky, Samaras, and Kopin[38] described a prototype mechanical device designed to control BP automatically by emulating portions of the baroreceptor reflex arc. Blood pressure was maintained at predetermined levels by the chronic intermittent infusion of norepinephrine for a period of 4 hours in two patients with multiple-system atrophy. Plasma NE levels doubled on standing, but no significant side effects were observed.

These investigators have continued testing this "sympathetic neural prosthesis" for 72 hours in two patients, who were able to carry out a normal schedule of activities and were asymptomatic.[39] Postprandial hypotension and sustained orthostatic hypotension did not occur. There appeared to be a reduction in sensitivity to NE. Clearly, further rigorous studies of this or similar devices is warranted.

REFERENCES

1. Bannister, R: *Treatment of progressive autonomic failure.* In Bannister, R (ed): *Autonomic Failure.* Oxford University Press, Oxford, 1983, pp 316–334.
2. Bevan, DR: *Shy-Drager syndrome: A review and description of the anesthetic management.* Anesthesia 31:866–873, 1979.
3. Malan, MD and Crago, RR: *Anaesthetic considerations in idiopathic orthostatic hypotension and the Shy-Drager syndrome.* Can Anaesth Soc J 26:322-327, 1979.
4. Maclean, AR and Allen, EV: *Orthostatic hypotension and orthostatic tachycardia: Treatment with the "head-up" bed.* JAMA 115:2162–2167, 1940.
5. Bannister, R, Ardill, L, and Fentem, P: *Defective autonomic control of blood vessels in idiopathic orthostatic hypotension.* Brain 90:725–746, 1967.
6. Bannister, R, Sever, P, and Gross, M: *Cardiovascular reflexes and biochemical responses in progressive autonomic failure.* Brain 100:327–344, 1977.
7. Sheps, SG: *Use of an elastic garment in the treatment of orthostatic hypotension.* Cardiology 61[Suppl I]: 271–279, 1976.
8. Schatz, IJ: *Orthostatic hypotension: II. Clinical diagnosis, testing and treatment.* Arch Intern Med 144:1037–1041, 1984.
9. Raab, W, Humphreys, RJ, and Lepeschkin, F: *Potentiation of pressor effects of norepinephrine and epinephrine in man by desoxycorticosterone acetate.* J Clin Invest 29:1397, 1950.
10. Davies, B: *Adrenergic receptors in automatic failure.* In Bannister, R (ed): *Autonomic Failure.* Oxford University Press, Oxford, 1983, pp 174–200.
11. Schatz, IJ, Miller, MJ, and Frame, B: *Corticosteroids in the management of orthostatic hypotension.* Cardiology 61[Suppl I]:280–289, 1976.

12. Mathias, C: Unpublished observations.

13. Bannister, R, Ardill, L, and Fentem, P: *An assessment of various methods of treatment of idiopathic orthostatic hypotension.* Q J Med 38:377–395, 1967.

14. Schirger, A, et al: *Midodrine—A new agent in the management of idiopathic orthostatic hypotension and Shy-Drager syndrome.* Proc Staff Meet Mayo Clin 56:429–433, 1981.

15. Thomas, JE, et al: *Orthostatic hypotension.* Mayo Clin Proc 56:117–125, 1981.

16. Diamond, MA, Murray, RH, and Schmid, PG: *Idiopathic postural hypotension; physiologic observations and report of a new mode of therapy.* J Clin Invest 49:1341–1348, 1970.

17. Mellander, S and Nordenfelt, I: *Comparative effects of dihydroergotamine and noradrenaline on resistance, exchange and capacity functions in the peripheral circulation.* Clin Sci 31:183–201, 1970.

18. Chobanian, AV, et al: *Treatment of chronic orthostatic hypotension with ergotamine.* Circulation 67:602–609, 1983.

19. Nordenfelt, I and Mellander, S: *Central haemodynamic effects of dihydroergotamine in patients with orthostatic hypotension.* Acta Med Scand 191:115–120, 1972.

20. Henry, PD and Yokoyama, M: *Supersensitivity of atherosclerotic rabbit aorta to ergonovine: Mediation by a serotonergic mechanism.* J Clin Invest 66:306–309, 1980.

21. Muller-Schweinitzer, E and Brundell, J: *Enhanced prostaglandin synthesis contributes to the venoconstrictor activity of ergotamine.* Blood Vessels 12:193–196, 1975.

22. Jenning, G, Esler, M, and Holmes, R: *Treatment of orthostatic hypotension with dihydroergotamine.* Br Med J 11:307–308, 1979.

23. Bobik, A, et al: *Low oral bioavailability of dihydroergotamine and first-pass extraction in patients with orthostatic hypotension.* Clin Pharmacol Ther 30:673–679, 1981.

24. Kochar, MS and Itskovitz, HD: *Treatment of idiopathic orthostatic hypotension (Shy-Drager syndrome) with indomethacin.* Lancet 1:1011–1014, 1978.

25. Abate, G, et al: *Effects of indomethacin on postural hypotension in parkinsonism.* Br Med J 2:1466–1468, 1979.

26. Davies, B, et al: *The pressor actions of noradrenaline and an-*

giotensin II in chronic autonomic failure treated with indomethacin. Br J Clin Pharmacol 10:223–229, 1980.

27. Abboud, FW and Eckstein, JW: *Active reflex vasodilatation in man.* Fed Proc 25:1611–1617, 1966.

28. Irving, MH, et al: *Effects of beta adrenergic blockade on plasma catecholamines in exercise.* Nature 248:531–533, 1974.

29. Chobanian, AV, et al: *Use of propranolol in the treatment of idiopathic orthostatic hypotension.* Trans Assoc Am Physicians 90:324–334, 1977.

30. Man in't Veld, AJ and Schalekamp, MADH: *Pindolol acts as beta-adrenoceptor agonist in orthostatic hypotension: Therapeutic implications.* Br Med J 282:929–931, 1981.

31. Davidson, AC and Smith, SE: *Pindolol in orthostatic hypotension.* Br Med J 282:1704(c), 1981.

32. Davies, B, et al: *Pindolol in postural hypotension; the cause for caution.* Lancet 2:982–983, 1981.

33. Man in't Veld, AJ, Boomsma, F, and Schalekamp, MADH: *Effects of β adrenoceptor agonists and antagonists in patients with peripheral autonomic neuropathy.* Br J Clin Pharmacol 13:3675–3745, 1982.

34. Robertson, D, et al: *Clonidine raises blood pressure in severe idiopathic orthostatic hypotension.* Am J Med 74:193–200, 1983.

35. Kuchel, O, et al: *Treatment of severe orthostatic hypotension by metoclopramide.* Ann Intern Med 93:841–843, 1980.

36. Moss, AJ, Galser, W, and Topol, E: *Atrial tachypacing in the treatment of a patient with primary orthostatic hypotension.* N Engl J Med 302:1456–1457, 1980.

37. Stackpoole, PW and Robertson, D: *Combination H_1 and H_2 receptor anagonist therapy in diabetic autonomic neuropathy.* South Med J 75:634–635, 1982.

38. Polinsky, RJ, Samaras, GM, and Kopin, IJ: *Sympathetic neural prosthesis for managing orthostatic hypotension.* Lancet 1:901–904, 1983.

39. Polinsky, RJ: Personal communication.

40. Frewin, DB and Bartholomeusz, FD: *Sea water: A novel self-medication for orthostatic hypotension.* Med J Aust 2:521–522, 1983.

41. Goovaerts, J, et al: *Effect of prenalterol on orthostatic hypoten-*

sion in the Shy-Drager syndrome. Br Med J 288:817–818, 1984.

42. Onrot, J, et al: *Hemodynamic and humoral effects of caffeine in autonomic failure.* N Engl J Med 313:549–554, 1985.

43. Ricci, DR et al: *Role of tachycardia as an inotropic stimulus in man.* J Clin Invest 63:695–703, 1979.

44. Kristinsson, A: *Programmed atrial pacing for orthostatic hypotension.* Acta Med Scand 214:79–83, 1983.

CHAPTER 7

ILLUSTRATIVE CASES

CASE 1: ORTHOSTATIC HYPOTENSION INDUCED BY DRUGS IN AN ELDERLY PATIENT

CASE 2: MITRAL VALVE PROLAPSE, AND SYMPATHICOTONIC ORTHOSTATIC HYPOTENSION

CASE 3: DIABETIC NEUROPATHY

CASE 4: MULTIPLE-SYSTEM ATROPHY (SHY-DRAGER SYNDROME)

CASE 5: IDIOPATHIC ORTHOSTATIC HYPOTENSION

CASE 6: AMYLOID NEUROPATHY

CASE 7: CAROTID SINUS OBLITERATION

CASE 8: MULTIPLE-SYSTEM ATROPHY (SHY-DRAGER SYNDROME)

The goal of this chapter is to integrate some of the material described heretofore by citing relevant examples from my personal clinical experience. Each case description was selected to underscore important points made in preceding chapters.

CASE 1: ORTHOSTATIC HYPOTENSION INDUCED BY DRUGS IN AN ELDERLY PATIENT

A 76-year-old retired schoolteacher was seen by her physician because of three "drop attacks" in the past 2 months. These were characterized by the sudden onset of loss of consciousness, preceded by vague feelings of a poorly described sensation of numbness in the hands and feet and an inability to focus her eyes. Each spell occurred while she was standing: one on first getting up in the morning, and the other two while she had been busy preparing a meal in the kitchen. Examination was unremarkable except for the presence of a recumbent blood pressure in the left arm of 160/95, and an upright blood pressure of 110/70. Ventricular rate was 75 supine and 95 standing. Neurologic examination was normal.

The patient had been receiving lorazepam (Ativan) in a dosage of 2 mg twice daily for the past 2 months and prazosin (Minipress) 1 mg twice daily for the past 3 months.

An organic cause for the orthostatic hypotension was thought to be highly unlikely, for two reasons: there was no evidence on examination of neurologic disease, and the cardioaccelerator (sympathetic) response was normal (heart rate rise of 20 beats per minute on standing). Because the patient was receiving at least two agents (lorazepam and prazosin) that could lead to drug-induced orthostatic hypotension, both were discontinued.

After 2 weeks, the recumbent blood pressure was 160/100 and the upright blood pressure was 130/80. Clearly, orthostatic hypotension was present, perhaps on the basis of diminished baroreceptor responsiveness seen in the aged. This probably was enhanced by the addition of the tranquilizer and antihypertensive agents. This synergism reduced the responsiveness of the autonomic nervous system to sympathetic and/or catecholamine influences, sufficient to induce significant symptoms of cerebral hypoxia.

Any patient who is receiving tranquilizers or antihypertensive drugs and presents with symptoms and signs of orthostatic hypotension must be considered to have drug-induced hypotension until proved otherwise. This is particularly true in elderly people, a substantial percentage of whom have physiologic diminution of the baroreceptor response and of autonomic reflexes.

If therapy for supine hypertension is thought to be necessary in the elderly, then care must be used in selecting a compound that will not induce orthostatic hypotension. This is not always easily done, since there is no way to predict which patients will have an adequate normotensive response to antihypertensive agents in the supine position, but not also react with an excessive blood pressure drop when standing. In my experience, small doses of beta-blocking drugs are probably best in this regard, but the cost of such therapy includes reduced mental acuity in many elderly patients.

CASE 2: MITRAL VALVE PROLAPSE, AND SYMPATHICOTONIC ORTHOSTATIC HYPOTENSION

A 28-year-old housewife had had increasing and progressive symptoms of fatigue, vague anterior chest pains, dizziness, and lightheadedness, particularly when she stood up. These were accompanied by symptoms of breathlessness and anxiety. A diagnosis of mitral valve prolapse had been made 3 years previously, on the basis of the presence of a loud systolic click with a following late systolic murmur. This was confirmed by two-dimensional echocardiography. The patient complained of occasional episodes of palpitations, but these had never been documented. She had been given various tranquilizing agents by her physician but without any apparent improvement in her subjective symptoms. Physical examination disclosed a thin-chested woman of moderate height with a systolic click and a late systolic murmur. The recumbent blood pressure was 115/75 with a pulse of 84 beats per minute. The blood pressure on standing was 90/65 with a pulse rate of 110 beats per minute. The patient complained of faintness and a "fluttery" sensation in the chest upon standing, and became pale and began to sweat.

Excessive sympathetic discharge on standing was obvious in this patient; a disproportionate tachycardia, together with pallor and sweating, indicates increased sympathetic tone. The accompanying orthostatic hypotension clearly reflected autonomic instability, since a normal response to sympathetic hyperactivity would be peripheral arterial constriction and increased cardiac inotropic activity, both of which would lead to an elevation of arterial pressure.

The patient responded remarkably to the administration of 20 mg of propranolol three times daily. After 1 month of such therapy, the recumbent blood pressure was 105/80 with a heart rate of 60 beats per minute, and the standing blood pressure was 100/65 with a heart rate of 75 beats per minute, and the symptoms were markedly diminished.

A substantial minority of patients with mitral valve prolapse have autonomic instability, manifested by orthostatic dizziness and vague symptoms of fatigue and anxiety. Sympathicotonic orthostatic hypotension (hypotension with excessive tachycardia, pallor, and sweating on standing) can be demonstrated in most. Fortunately, treatment with beta-adrenergic blockers is often beneficial.

CASE 3: DIABETIC NEUROPATHY

A 52-year-old patient with Type II diabetes mellitus had symptoms of peripheral neuropathy for approximately 15 years. These were characterized by paresthesia of the feet and toes and, recently, occasional episodes of lancinating nocturnal pain in the right foot. Over the past 3 years, he had noticed gradually increasing impotence; for 6 months, there had been occasional episodes of nocturnal diarrhea. For the past 3 weeks, he had four discrete episodes of marked lightheadedness and dizziness upon standing; these occurred when he first got up in the morning to urinate. On one occasion, he was certain that he was about to faint, and had to slump to the floor. He took vitamin supplements and 38 units of NPH insulin every morning. He stated that diabetes control had been good; his last fasting blood glucose was 143 mg percent.

Examination revealed a recumbent blood pressure of 130/80 with a ventricular rate of 84 beats per minute. On standing, the blood pressure fell to 75/50 with a pulse rate of 90 beats per minute, and he became lightheaded. Neurologic examination revealed the stigmata of peripheral sensory neuropathy, together with some diminution of deep tendon reflexes in the legs. Clearly, a diagnosis of autonomic dysfunction and autonomic neuropathy in this patient was warranted. The impotence, symptoms of paresthesia, recent orthostatic hypotension, nocturnal diarrhea, and lack of appropriate positive chronotropic response to standing all indicated sympathetic insufficiency. Although tests of autonomic function would have been of interest, it is doubtful that knowledge of their results would contribute meaningfully to management.

Physical measures were first instituted: a waist-length (Jobst) leotard with 40 mm Hg of pressure at the ankles was fitted. The patient began to sleep with the head of the bed elevated, and learned to rise very slowly in the morning. After 3 months of such therapy, he had no symptoms of orthostasis, although a drop in standing blood pressure could be demonstrated on examination (from 120/70 to 90/60). He has been maintained on physical measures alone with a liberalized salt intake for the past 18 months.

This case demonstrates the utility of physical measures in the initial therapy for patients with orthostatic hypotension. The physician must emphasize the importance of wearing a pressure gradient support, and of sleeping with the head of the bed elevated. Although orthostatic hypotension was still present in this patient, physical measures had raised the mean arterial pressure sufficiently to exceed that threshold of cerebral perfusion below which symptoms of hypoxia developed. It is important to emphasize that the major objective of therapy is to obviate symptoms of cerebral hypoxia.

CASE 4: MULTIPLE-SYSTEM ATROPHY (SHY-DRAGER SYNDROME)

A 32-year-old housewife had symptoms of unsteadiness and clumsiness since age 18. These had gradually progressed so that at present she needs to walk with the aid of a cane and usually holds on to something while she is standing in the kitchen preparing meals. Dizziness, lightheadedness, and occasional syncope first began about 5 years ago, particularly upon first arising in the morning. These now occur perhaps three or four times a month, and can be aborted by sitting down or by slumping. Striking hoarseness of the voice was first noted about 3 years ago and has become progressive. She has no symptoms of incontinence but does complain of considerable "gas."

Examination revealed a very thin, rather emaciated woman who had a wide-based gait and signs of both extrapyramidal and cerebellar dysfunction. Babinski responses were present bilaterally. The blood pressure was 100/60 recumbent, with a ventricular rate of 84, and 60/? upright with a ventricular rate of 88. Examination of her vocal cords revealed paralysis of the vocal abductors. Previous neurologic investigations had revealed no signs of intracranial masses. Electroencephalogram was normal.

Currently, the patient is maintained with a waist-length Jobst support, the head of her bed elevated at 20 degrees at night, a very liberal salt intake, 9-alpha-fludrocortisone (0.6 mg daily), ephedrine sulfate (25 mg three times daily), and pindolol (10 mg twice daily).

She has adhered to this program for approximately 1½ years without any worsening of her symptoms of orthostatic hypotension. Her neurologic deficits, however, may have progressed somewhat over this period.

This case is an excellent example of multiple-system atrophy, which often is progressive, insidious, and essentially untreatable. Nevertheless, this patient still maintains function, since her major disability of orthostatic hypotension has been treated by appropriate use of physical and pharmacologic measures. The usual mainstay of therapy is the use of 9-alpha-fludrocortisone. Frequent evaluation for supine hypertension, hypokalemia, and edema accumulation is mandatory. This patient did develop hypokalemia approximately 6 months ago, which responded to appropriate potassium supplements. Although her prognosis is guarded, she is able to maintain a useful and productive life, in great part because of the positive and supportive attitude of her family, and substantial amounts of reassurance from her physician.

Unfortunately, the natural course of multiple-system atrophy (Shy-Drager syndrome) may be more rapidly downhill in some cases. The patient cited above developed orthostatic hypotension well after the first clinical signs and symptoms of neurologic disease appeared; in some, however, neurologic impairment may be such that a combination of severe orthostatic hypotension and neurologic deficits become intractable and untreatable.

CASE 5: IDIOPATHIC ORTHOSTATIC HYPOTENSION

A 46-year-old man first began having symptoms of inability to develop and maintain an erection about 3 years ago. He sought advice from a urologist who, after extensive investigation, concluded that the impotence was psychogenic; subsequent psychotherapy was ineffective. About 18 months ago, he returned to the urologist because of increasing incontinence. He was finally referred to a general internist who measured a recumbent blood pressure in the right arm of 130/90 and a ventricular rate of 84, and an upright blood pressure of 70/40 and a ventricular rate of 84. Examination was otherwise unremarkable; in particular, there were no neurologic deficits that could be detected.

The patient was referred to me with the following questions:

1. Should the orthostatic hypotension be treated?
2. What further investigations were required?
3. What was the patient's prognosis?

On examination, the supine and upright blood pressures were as above. Careful neurologic investigation revealed no signs of pyramidal, extrapyramidal, cerebellar, or peripheral neuropathic disease.

Since the patient had no symptoms of orthostatic hypotension, nor of angina pectoris, management specifically aimed at improving blood pressure on standing was not warranted. No evidence is available to suggest that improving the hemodynamics in patients with idiopathic orthostatic hypotension makes any difference to their neurologic disease.

Although extensive laboratory investigations could have been performed, it is arguable whether they were necessary. The reasons for documenting the presence or absence of detectable neurologic disease is to provide a baseline for longitudinal follow-up of the patient, so that if new neurologic signs emerge, then the differentiation between multiple-system atrophy and idiopathic orthostatic hypotension can be made. In my opinion, such differentiation is probably not necessary so early in the course of the illness, unless the patient insists on having as precise an idea as to prognosis as the physician can provide. In general, longevity of patients with idiopathic orthostatic hypotension is better than for patients with multiple-system atrophy. Accordingly, some may wish to make long-term plans on the basis of this knowledge. Most, however, are satisfied with the knowledge that careful and reassuring follow-up by their physicians will provide ample opportunity for prognostic statements.

In this case, I chose not to do any extensive neurologic investigations but to merely follow the patient. For the past 18 months, there has been no progression of neurologic signs or symptoms nor any worsening of orthostatic hypotension. The impotence and incontinence are managed by the urologist. It is important for the patient to know, however, that his general physician is available for potential problems if they should emerge. Since patients with idiopathic orthostatic hypotension may have a stable course, appropriate reassurance is mandatory. Even if the orthostatic hypotension worsens and creates symptoms of cerebral hypoxia, there is every likelihood that these may be managed successfully by a combination of physical and pharmacologic measures.

CASE 6: AMYLOID NEUROPATHY

A 67-year-old man had a 4-month history of severe nocturnal diarrhea. Signs of sensory and motor neuropathy appeared, followed very closely by rather dramatic symptoms of orthostatic hypotension. Rectal biopsy revealed amyloidosis.

The patient was referred for management of his severe orthostasis. Recumbent blood pressure was 110/70 with a ventricular rate of 74; blood pressure standing was 70/? with a ventricular rate of 76. The patient could not stand without support for longer than 30 seconds. The diagnosis of severe amyloid neuropathy was obvious. Therapy with Jobst waist-length leotard, sleeping with the head of the bed elevated, and liberal salt intake was instituted. An initial dose of 0.1 mg of 9-alpha-fludrocortisone was started; this was increased by 0.1-mg increments every 5 days to 0.4 mg. At the end of 1 month, the standing blood pressure was 80/60, but symptoms of cerebral hypoxia persisted. Increasing the dosage of fludrocortisone to 0.5 mg daily produced supine hypertension (210/120) and congestive heart failure. Reduction of the fludrocortisone by 0.1 mg to 0.4 mg daily eliminated these complications. The serial addition of various other medications, including indomethacin, ephedrine sulfate, metamphetamine, pindolol, and clonidine, was not efficacious. Symptoms became so severe that the patient had to be maintained at bed rest because he could not get up to go to the bathroom.

Progressive orthostatic hypotension was manifested by a drop in blood pressure when the patient sat up at 75 degrees: recumbent blood pressure was maintained at 100/60 but dropped to 70 systolic during this position.

The patient died of pneumonia 4 weeks after admission to a skilled nursing facility.

In my experience, amyloidosis creates the most difficult management problems in patients with orthostatic hypotension. The above case is an example of an intractable and malignant disease for which no therapeutic strategies were successful.

CASE 7: CAROTID SINUS OBLITERATION

A 72-year-old man had a nasopharyngeal squamous cell carcinoma excised 18 months previously. Extensive regional node metastases had been present, and the patient was treated with x-ray therapy postoperatively. During the past month, physical examination revealed the recurrence of a very firm mass over the entire right neck. At the same time, the patient has had symptoms of marked dizziness upon standing. The recumbent blood pressure was 130/90 with a ventricular rate of 84; standing blood pressure fell to 70/40 with a ventricular rate of 96 beats per minute. The patient was treated with a waist-length leotard and 0.2 mg of 9-alpha-fludrocortisone daily. Orthostatic symptoms improved, and the patient underwent chemotherapy for his recurrent carcinoma.

In this patient, the afferent limb of the baroreceptor reflex arc is involved; extensive destruction of the right carotid sinus has interfered with afferent signals to integrating centers in the brain. The orthostatic hypotension is relatively easily managed by the usual methods, permitting palliative therapy for his regional metastases.

CASE 8: MULTIPLE-SYSTEM ATROPHY (SHY-DRAGER SYNDROME)

A 46-year-old mechanic first developed hoarseness about 4 years ago. He saw an otorhinolaryngologist, who found bilateral vocal abductor cord paralysis of unknown cause. Extensive neurologic investigation was unremarkable. About 2 years ago, the patient first began having clumsiness of gait and rigidity of his extremities. Neurologic investigation at that time disclosed the signs of parkinsonism. About 6 months ago, he first began having symptoms of dizziness when getting up in the morning to urinate. Three months ago, he began complaining of symptoms of incontinence.

Physical examination revealed the facies of parkinsonism, with marked cogwheeling and rigidity of the extremities. The patient's voice had a peculiar "breathy" sound. Recumbent blood pressure was 110/70 with a ventricular rate of 80; upright blood pressure fell to 70/? with a ventricular rate of 82 per minute. Recumbent plasma norepinephrine levels were 264 pg/ml; after 1 minute of being upright, these levels were 312 pg/ml.

The patient responded well to a program consisting of sleeping with the head of the bed elevated, a waist-length pressure-gradient (Jobst) support, 0.3 mg of 9-alpha-fludrocortisone daily, and indomethacin 25 mg three times daily. At present, he has no symptoms of orthostasis; the standing blood pressure is 90/70; the recumbent blood pressure is 140/100. Fasting blood glucose and serum potassium are normal.

The presence of vocal abductor cord paralysis is an important clue to the presence of multiple-system atrophy. In order to confirm this diagnosis, however, plasma norepinephrine measurements were made; in patients with multiple-system atrophy there are usually normal levels of plasma norepinephrine while recumbent, which do not increase appropriately upon standing. In normal subjects, there is a twofold to fourfold increase in plasma norepinephrine when upright. Patients with idiopathic orthostatic hypotension have extremely low levels of plasma norepinephrine when supine, which do not increase when the patient stands.

Thus, differentiation between idiopathic orthostatic hypotension and multiple-system atrophy may be made on the basis of the level of recumbent plasma norepinephrine levels.

The natural course of multiple-system atrophy is quite variable. Patients often present first with neurologic defects; symptoms of reduced cerebral arterial perfusion appear later. Stabilizing the hemodynamic consequences of orthostatic hypotension will obviously improve day-to-day living; nevertheless, if other manifestations of neurologic disease progress, then impairment and disability will follow. Remissions, exacerbations, and a generally unpredictable course are the rule, however. Occasional patients may have an inexorable and progressively downhill history, while others may stabilize for months or even years at an acceptable level of functioning. The primary-care physician must act as a "gatekeeper" in coordinating the efforts of the neurologist, urologist, occupational therapist, physical therapist, and members of the family in making maximum use of the patient's functional capabilities.

EPILOGUE

Although the prevalence of orthostatic hypotension is unknown, on occasion most primary-care physicians will be faced with the diagnosis and management of this syndrome. Because patients have symptoms and signs that cross conventional interdisciplinary lines, it often becomes the responsibility of a family physician or general internist to provide overall direction for ongoing management. In order to do so intelligently, the clinician needs access to a single source of information about postural hypotension, which was the goal of this monograph.

Specialists have patients referred for specific problems related to those disorders in which postural hypotension may play some role. For example, hoarseness may be the presenting symptom of multiple-system atrophy, and urinary incontinence often is the first sign of idiopathic orthostatic hypotension. Thus, awareness that these symptoms may reflect a systemic disorder is mandatory for otorhinolaryngologists and urologists. Cardiologists provide consultation on patients sent for advice concerning inability to maintain blood pressure when upright, and neurologists, of course, have to distinguish among multiple-system atrophy, idiopathic orthostatic hypotension, idiopathic parkinsonism, and the various peripheral neuropathies as the fundamental cause of hypotension in patients with specific neurologic deficits.

I have attempted to describe the normal circulatory mechanisms that operate to maintain adequate blood pressure on standing, and also how disturbances of this delicate homeostasis induce significant defects in blood pressure control. The lengthy and ubiquitous list of both functional and organic causes of orthostatic hypotension should make the clinician sensitized to these possibilities. For instance, baroreceptor deficiency in the elderly may or may not play an important role in inducing dizzy spells, but it is essential for all clinicians to be aware of the relatively high prevalence of postural hypotension in this age group, no matter what the ultimate cause.

The most important of the permanent forms of orthostatic hypotension clearly are related to neurologic disease. Since some confusion may exist about the pathophysiologic and clinical separation of neurologic causes of orthostatic hypotension, I have included a detailed discussion of the differences among multiple-system atrophy (Shy-Drager syndrome), idiopathic orthostatic hypotension, and idiopathic parkinsonism. Newer data concerning the pharmacologic and biochemical distinction among these syndromes have been emphasized. Similarly, the recent advances in understanding the relationship between excessive sympathetic discharge, as is seen in sympathicotonic orthostatic hypotension, with or without mitral valve prolapse, have received careful attention.

Although the diagnosis may be reached by the simple application of common sense and good clinical skills, sometimes autonomic nervous system testing becomes necessary in order to detect differences and tailor pharmacologic therapy. Similarly, management strategies differ from patient to patient, but the underlying goal is to achieve maximum day-to-day mobility. This is best accomplished by capitalizing on those physiologic (head-up tilt, added dietary sodium), physical (pressure-gradient supports), and pharmacologic (various drugs) means available to us. To do this successfully requires a thorough understanding of the benefits and risks of these measures. The final outcome is a patient who continues to lead a useful and productive life.

INDEX

A t following a page number indicates a table. A page number in *italics* indicates a figure.

ADRENAL insufficiency, orthostatic hypotension and, 20

Adrenergic blockers, management of orthostatic hypotension and, 105–107

Adrenergic receptors, postsynaptic, neurogenic orthostatic hypotension and, 61

Afferent function tests, clinical diagnosis of orthostatic hypotension and
- amyl nitrate inhalation, 82
- heart rate response to standing, 81–82
- phenylephrine hydrochloride injection, 83
- vasopressin response to standing, 83

Afferent lesions, neurogenic orthostatic hypotension and, 27–28

Aging, orthostatic hypotension and, 16–17

Amyl nitrate inhalation, clinical diagnosis of orthostatic hypotension and, 82

Amyloid neuropathy, case study of, orthostatic hypotension and, 120–121

Anorexia nervosa, orthostatic hypotension and, 17

Antidiuretic hormone. *See also* Arginine vasopressin
- neurogenic orthostatic hypotension and, 61–62

Arginine vasopressin
maintenance of normal blood pressure upon standing and, 8
neurogenic orthostatic hypotension and, 61–62
Arithmetic under stress, clinical diagnosis of orthostatic hypotension and, 84
Arterial perfusion, inadequate, clinical diagnosis of orthostatic hypotension and symptoms of, 69–70
Arteriolar constriction, reflex, maintenance of normal blood pressure upon standing and, 2–6
baroreceptor reflex arc and, *4,* 4–5
postsynaptic sympathetic varicosity and, *5,* 5
Asthenic habitus, orthostatic hypotension and, 15
Atrial tachypacing, management of orthostatic hypotension and, 107–108
Atrophy, multiple-system. *See also* Multiple-system atrophy
neurogenic orthostatic hypotension and, 35–38
pathology and pathogenesis of, 38–39, *40,* 41
AVP. *See* Arginine vasopressin
Autonomic dysfunction, symptoms of, clinical diagnosis of orthostatic hypotension and, 70–72
Autonomic function tests, clinical diagnosis of orthostatic hypotension and, 78, 79t
modified noninvasive Valsalva maneuver, 81
Valsalva maneuver, 78, *80,* 80–81

BED rest, orthostatic hypotension and, 15–16
Blood pressure
drugs that affect, 19–20
low. *See* Hypotension
normal, maintenance of, upon standing, 1–2, 2t, *3*
cerebral blood flow and, 9–10
hormonal responses and, 8
increase in heart rate and, 6–8, *7*
reflex arteriolar constriction and, 2–6, *4, 5*
reflex venous constriction and, 6
respiratory and muscle changes and, 10
Blood volume, reduced effective circulatory, orthostatic hypo-

tension due to, 18–19

CAFFEINE, management of orthostatic hypotension and, 108

Carotid sinus obliteration, case study of orthostatic hypotension and, 121–122

Case studies of orthostatic hypotension, 113–114
- amyloid neuropathy, 120–121
- carotid sinus obliteration, 121–122
- diabetic neuropathy, 116–117
- drug-induced orthostatic hypotension in an elderly patient, 114–115
- idiopathic orthostatic hypotension, 119–120
- mitral valve prolapse and sympathicotonic orthostatic hypotension, 115–116
- multiple-system atrophy (Shy-Drager syndrome), 117–119, 122–124

Catecholamine studies, plasma, neurogenic orthostatic hypotension and, 57, 58t, 59

Central disorders, neurogenic orthostatic hypotension and, 29
- idiopathic parkinsonism, 29–30
- miscellaneous causes, 30–31
- Riley-Day syndrome (familial dysautonomia), 30

Central function tests, clinical diagnosis of orthostatic hypotension and, 83–84

Cerebral blood flow, maintenance of normal blood pressure upon standing and, 9–10

Clinical diagnosis of orthostatic hypotension, 68t, 68–69
- clinical use of autonomic function testing and, 87–88
- laboratory investigations and, 76–78
- patient history and, 72–74, 73t
- physical examination and, 73t, 74–76
- symptoms of autonomic dysfunction and, 70–72
- symptoms of inadequate arterial perfusion and, 69–70
- tests of afferent function and
  - amyl nitrate inhalation, 82
  - heart rate response to standing, 81–82
  - phenylephrine hydrochloride injection, 83
  - vasopressin response to standing, 83

Clinical diagnosis of orthostatic hypotension—*continued*
  tests of autonomic function and, 78, 79t
    modified noninvasive Valsalva maneuver, 81
    Valsalva maneuver, 78, *80,* 80–81
  tests of central function and, 83–84
  tests of efferent function and
    invasive
      norepinephrine infusion, 86–87
      tyramine infusion, 86
    noninvasive
      arithmetic under stress, 84
      cold pressor test, 84
      epinephrine instillation into the eye, 85
      plasma norepinephrine levels, 85–86
      sweat tests, 84–85
Clonidine, management of orthostatic hypotension and, 107
Cold pressor test, clinical diagnosis of orthostatic hypotension and, 84
Constriction
  reflex arteriolar, maintenance of normal blood pressure upon standing and, 2–6
    baroreceptor reflex arc and, *4,* 4–5
    postsynaptic sympathetic varicosity and, *5,* 5
  reflex venous, maintenance of normal blood pressure upon standing and, 6
Counterpressure support garment, 95, *96,* 97

DERANGEMENTS
  functional, orthostatic hypotension due to, 13, 14t
    inadequate postural adjustment and
      aging and, 16–17
      asthenic habitus with poorly developed musculature and, 15
      bed rest and/or space flight and, 15–16
      miscellaneous causes and, 17–18
      physical exertion and, 15
    miscellaneous causes and, 20–21
    pharmacologic agents and, 19–20
    reduced effective circulatory blood volume and, 18–19
  organic, orthostatic hypotension due to, 26
    defects in peripheral vasculature and
      congenital defect in norepinephrine release and, 48
      hyperbradykininism and, 47–48

neurogenic orthostatic hypotension and, 26–27, 27t, 28t
afferent lesions and, 27–28
central disorders and, 29
idiopathic parkinsonism, 29–30
miscellaneous causes, 30–31
Riley-Day syndrome (familial dysautonomia), 30
disorders primarily affecting sympathetic chain and postganglionic nerves and
diabetes mellitus, 44–45
miscellaneous neuropathies, 45–47
efferent defects and 31, 32t–33t, 34
idiopathic orthostatic hypotension, 34
multiple-system atrophy (Shy-Drager syndrome), 35–38
miscellaneous lesions in the spinal cord and, 44
orthostatic hypotension and mitral valve prolapse and, 42–44, 43t
orthostatic hypotension associated with excessive sympathetic discharge (sympathicotonic orthostatic hypotension) and, 41–42
pathology and pathogenesis of multiple-system atrophy and idiopathic orthostatic hypotension and, 38–39, *40,* 41
Diabetes mellitus, orthostatic hypotension and, 44–45
Diabetic neuropathy, case study of orthostatic hypotension and, 116–117
Diagnosis, clinical, of orthostatic hypotension, 68t, 68–69
clinical use of autonomic function testing and, 87–88
laboratory investigations and, 76–78
patient history and, 72–74, 73t
physical examination and, 73t, 74–76
symptoms of autonomic dysfunction and, 70–72
symptoms of inadequate arterial perfusion and, 69–70
tests of afferent function and
amyl nitrate inhalation, 82
heart rate response to standing, 81–82
phenylephrine hydrochloride injection, 83

Diagnosis, clinical, of orthostatic hypotension—*continued*
- vasopressin response to standing, 83
- tests of autonomic function and, 78, 79t
  - modified noninvasive Valsalva maneuver, 81
  - Valsalva maneuver, 78, *80,* 80–81
- tests of central function and, 83–84
- tests of efferent function and
  - invasive
    - norepinephrine infusion, 86–87
    - tyramine infusion, 86
  - noninvasive
    - arithmetic under stress, 84
    - cold pressor test, 84
    - epinephrine instillation into the eye, 85
    - plasma norepinephrine levels, 85–86
    - sweat tests, 84–85

Dihydroergotamine. *See* Ergot derivatives

Dopamine, infusion of, orthostatic hypotension and, 62–63

Drug-induced orthostatic hypotension, case study of, in elderly patient, 114–115

Drugs that affect blood pressure, 19–20

Dysautonomia, familial. *See* Riley-Day syndrome

Dysfunction, autonomic, symptoms of, clinical diagnosis of orthostatic hypotension and, 70–72

EFFERENT defects, neurogenic orthostatic hypotension and, 31, 32t–33t, 34
- idiopathic orthostatic hypotension, 34
- multiple-system atrophy (Shy-Drager syndrome), 35–38

Efferent function tests, clinical diagnosis of orthostatic hypotension and
- invasive
  - norepinephrine infusion, 86–87
  - tyramine infusion, 86
- noninvasive
  - arithmetic under stress, 84
  - cold pressor test, 84
  - epinephrine instillation into the eye, 85
  - plasma norepinephrine levels, 85–86
  - sweat tests, 84–85

Electrolyte disturbances, orthostatic hypotension and, 20

Enzyme measurements, neurogenic orthostatic hypotension and, 62

Ephedrine, management of orthostatic hypotension and, 100
Epinephrine, instillation into the eye, clinical diagnosis of orthostatic hypotension and, 85
Ergotamine tartrate. *See* Ergot derivatives
Ergot derivatives, management of orthostatic hypotension and, 102, 103t, 104t
Examination, physical, clinical diagnosis of orthostatic hypotension and, 73t, 74–76
Excessive sympathetic discharge, orthostatic hypotension and, 41–42
Exertion, physical, orthostatic hypotension and, 15

FAMILIAL dysautonomia. *See* Riley-Day syndrome
Fever, orthostatic hypotension and, 18
Fludrocortisone acetate, management of orthostatic hypotension and, 98–100, 99t, 100t
Functional derangements, orthostatic hypotension due to, 13, 14t
  inadequate postural adjustment and
    aging and, 16–17
    asthenic habitus with poorly developed musculature and, 15
    bed rest and/or space flight and, 15–16
    miscellaneous causes and, 17–18
    physical exertion and, 15
  miscellaneous causes and, 20–21
  pharmacologic agents and, 19–20
  reduced effective circulatory blood volume and, 18–19

GASTRECTOMY, orthostatic hypotension after, 17
General measures, management of orthostatic hypotension and, 93-94

HABITUS, asthenic, orthostatic hypotension and, 15
Head-up tilt at night, management of orthostatic hypotension and, 95
Heart rate
  increase in, maintenance of normal blood pressure upon standing and, *3*, 6–8, *7*

Heart rate—*continued*
response to standing, clinical diagnosis of orthostatic hypotension and, 81–82
History, patient, clinical diagnosis of orthostatic hypotension and, 72–74, 73t
Hormonal responses, maintenance of normal blood pressure upon standing and, 8
arginine vasopressin and, 8
renin-angiotensin-aldosterone system and, 8
vanillylmandelic acid and, 8
Hydroxyamphetamine, management of orthostatic hypotension and, 101
Hyperbradykininism, orthostatic hypotension and, 47–48
Hypotension, orthostatic
case studies of, 113–114
amyloid neuropathy, 120–121
carotid sinus obliteration, 121–122
diabetic neuropathy, 116–117
drug-induced orthostatic hypotension in an elederly patient, 114–115
idiopathic orthostatic hypotension, 119–120
mitral valve prolapse and sympathicotonic orthostatic hypotension, 115–116
multiple-system atrophy (Shy-Drager syndrome), 117–119, 122–124
clinical diagnosis of, 68t, 68–69
clinical use of autonomic function testing and, 87–88
laboratory investigations and, 76–78
patient history and, 72–74, 73t
physical examination and, 73t, 74–76
symptoms of autonomic dysfunction and, 70–72
symptoms of inadequate arterial perfusion and, 69–70
tests of afferent function and
amyl nitrate inhalation, 82
heart rate response to standing, 81–82
phenylephrine hydrochloride injection, 83
vasopressin response to standing, 83
tests of autonomic function and, 78, 79t
modified noninvasive Valsalva maneuver, 81
Valsalva maneuver, 78, *80,* 80–81
tests of central function and, 83–84

tests of efferent function
invasive
norepinephrine infusion, 86–87
tyramine infusion, 86
noninvasive
arithmetic under stress, 84
cold pressor test, 84
epinephrine instillation into the eye, 85
plasma norepinephrine levels, 85–86
sweat tests, 84–85
excessive sympathetic discharge and, 41–42
Hypotension, orthostatic
functional derangements and, 13, 14t
inadequate postural adjustment and aging and, 16–17
asthenic habitus with poorly developed musculature and, 15
bed rest and/or space flight and, 15–16
miscellaneous causes and, 17–18
physical exertion and, 15
miscellaneous causes and, 20–21
pharmacologic agents and, 19–20
reduced effective circulatory blood volume and, 18–19
idiopathic, 34
management of, 91–93, 92t
general measures for, 93–94
mechanical devices for, 108–109
pharmacologic measures for, 97–98, 98t
adrenergic blockers, 105–107
ergot derivatives, 102, 103t, 104t
fludrocortisone acetate, 98–100, 99t, 100t
miscellaneous agents, 107–108
prostaglandin inhibition, 105
vasopressors, 100–101
physical measures for
head-up tilt at night, 95
lower body external pressure, 95, *96*, 97
mitral valve prolapse and, 42–44, 43t
neurogenic, 26–27, 27t, 28t
afferent lesions and, 27–28
central disorders and, 29
idiopathic parkinsonism, 29–30
miscellaneous causes, 30–31
Riley-Day syndrome (familial dysautonomia), 30
defects in peripheral vasculature and
congenital defect in norepinephrine release and, 48

Hypotension, orthostatic—*continued*
hyperbradykininism and, 47–48
disorders primarily affecting sympathetic chain and postganglionic nerves and
diabetes mellitus, 44–45
miscellaneous neuropathies, 45–47
efferent defects and, 31, 32t–33t, 34
idiopathic orthostatic hypotension, 34
multiple-system atrophy (Shy-Drager syndrome), 35–38
miscellaneous lesions in the spinal cord and, 44
orthostatic hypotension and mitral valve prolapse and, 42–44, 43t
orthostatic hypotension associated with excessive sympathetic discharge (sympathicotonic orthostatic hypotension) and, 41–42
pathology and pathogenesis of multiple-system atrophy and idiopathic orthostatic hypotension and, 38–39, *40,* 41
pathophysiologic and pharmacologic investigations of, 55–57, *56*
antidiuretic hormone (arginine vasopressin) and, 61–62
enzyme measurements and, 62
plasma catecholamine studies and, 57, 58t, 59
postsynaptic adrenergic receptors and, 61
pressor agent infusions and, 59–61, 60t, 62–63
spinal cord lesions and, 44
sympathetic chain and postganglionic nerve disorders and
diabetes mellitus, 44–45
miscellaneous neuropathies, 45–47
Hypothyroidism, orthostatic hypotension and, 21

IDIOPATHIC orthostatic hypotension, 34
case study of, 119–120
Idiopathic parkinsonism, neurogenic orthostatic hypotension and, 29–30
Inadequate arterial perfusion, clinical diagnosis of orthostatic hypotension and symptoms of, 69–70
Insulin tolerance test, neuro-

genic orthostatic hypotension and, 63
Indomethacin, management of orthostatic hypotension and, 105
Infectious neuronitis, orthostatic hypotension and, 21
Isoproterenol, infusion of, neurogenic orthostatic hypotension and, 63

Labetalol, management of orthostatic hypotension and, 106
Laboratory investigations, clinical diagnosis of orthostatic hypotension and, 76–78
L-dopa, management of orthostatic hypotension and, 107
Lesions
- afferent, neurogenic orthostatic hypotension and, 27–28
- spinal cord, orthostatic hypotension and, 44

Lower body external pressure, management of orthostatic hypotension and, 95, *96*, 97

Malignancy, orthostatic hypotension and, 21
Management of orthostatic hypotension, 91–93, 92t
- general measures for, 93–94
- mechanical devices for, 108–109
- pharmacologic measures for, 97–98, 98t
  - adrenergic blockers, 105–107
  - ergot derivatives, 102, 103t, 104t
  - fludrocortisone acetate, 98–100, 99t, 100t
  - miscellaneous agents, 107–108
  - prostaglandin inhibition, 105
  - vasopressors, 100–101
- physical measures for
  - head-up tilt at night, 95
  - lower body external pressure, 95, *96*, 97

Marijuana, orthostatic hypotension after use of, 18
Mechanical devices, management of orthostatic hypotension and, 108–109
Methoxamine, infusion of, neurogenic orthostatic hypotension and, 63
3-Methoxy-4-hydroxymandelic acid. *See* Vanillylmandelic acid
Methylphenidate, management of orthostatic hypotension and, 101
Metoclopramide, management of orthostatic hypotension and, 107

Midodrine, management of orthostatic hypotension and, 100–101
Mitral valve prolapse
case study of sympathicotonic orthostatic hypotension and, 115–116
orthostatic hypotension and, 42–44, 43t
Muscle and respiratory changes, maintenance of normal blood pressure upon standing and, 10
Multiple-system atrophy
case study of orthostatic hypotension and, 117–119, 122–124
neurogenic orthostatic hypotension and, 35–38
pathology and pathogenesis of, 38–39, *40,* 41

NEURONITIS, infectious, orthostatic hypotension and, 21
Neuropathy
amyloid, case study of orthostatic hypotension and, 120–121
diabetic, case study of orthostatic hypotension and, 116–117
miscellaneous, orthostatic hypotension and, 45–47
Norepinephrine
congenital defect in release of, orthostatic hypotension and, 48
infusion of
clinical diagnosis of orthostatic hypotension and, 86–87
orthostatic hypotension and, 60–61, 60t
plasma levels of, 57, 58t, 59
clinical diagnosis of orthostatic hypotension and, 85–86
storage and release of, 55–57, *56*

ORGANIC derangements, orthostatic hypotension due to, 26
defects in peripheral vasculature and
congenital defect in norepinephrine release and, 48
hyperbradykininism and, 47–48
neurogenic orthostatic hypotension and, 26–27, 27t, 28t
afferent lesions and, 27–28
central disorders and, 29
idiopathic parkinsonism, 29–30
miscellaneous causes, 30–31
Riley-Day syndrome (familial dysautonomia), 30
disorders primarily affecting sympathetic chain and

postganglionic nerves and
diabetes mellitus, 44–45
miscellaneous neuropathies, 45–47
efferent defects and, 31, 32t–33t, 34
idiopathic orthostatic hypotension, 34
multiple-system atrophy (Shy-Drager syndrome), 35–38
miscellaneous lesions in the spinal cord and, 44
orthostatic hypotension and mitral valve prolapse and, 42–44, 43t
orthostatic hypotension associated with excessive sympathetic discharge (sympathicotonic orthostatic hypotension) and, 41–42
pathology and pathogenesis of multiple-system atrophy and idiopathic orthostatic hypotension and, 38–39, *40,* 41
Orthostatic hypotension
case studies of, 113–114
amyloid neuropathy, 120–121
carotid sinus obliteration, 121–122
diabetic neuropathy, 116–117
drug-induced orthostatic hypotension in an elderly patient, 114–115
idiopathic orthostatic hypotension, 119–120
mitral valve prolapse and sympathicotonic orthostatic hypotension, 115–116
multiple-system atrophy (Shy-Drager syndrome), 117–119, 122–124
clinical diagnosis of, 68t, 68–69
clinical use of autonomic function testing and, 87–88
laboratory investigations and, 76–78
patient history and, 72–74, 73t
physical examination and, 73t, 74–76
symptoms of autonomic dysfunction and, 70–72
symptoms of inadequate arterial perfusion and, 69–70
tests of afferent function and
amyl nitrate inhalation, 82
heart rate reponse to standing, 81–82
phenylephrine hydrochloride injection, 83
vasopressin response to standing, 83

Orthostatic hypotension—*continued*
tests of autonomic function and, 78, 79t
modified noninvasive Valsalva maneuver, 81
Valsalva maneuver, 78, *80,* 80–81
tests of central function and, 83–84
tests of efferent function and
invasive
norepinephrine infusion, 86–87
tyramine infusion, 86
noninvasive
arithmetic under stress, 84
cold pressor test, 84
epinephrine instillation into the eye, 85
plasma norepinephrine levels, 85–86
sweat tests, 84–85
defects in peripheral vasculature and
congenital defect in norepinephrine release and, 48
hyperbradykininism and, 47–48
excessive sympathetic discharge and, 41–42
functional derangements and, 13, 14t
inadequate postural adjustment and
aging and, 16–17
asthenic habitus with poorly developed musculature and, 15
bed rest and/or space flight and, 15–16
miscellaneous causes and, 17–18
physical exertion and, 15
miscellaneous causes and, 20–21
pharmacologic agents and, 19–20
reduced effective circulatory blood volume and, 18–19
idiopathic, 34
management of, 91–93, 92t
general measures for, 93–94
mechanical devices for, 108–109
pharmacologic measures for, 97–98, 98t
adrenergic blockers, 105–107
ergot derivatives, 102, 103t, 104t
fludrocortisone acetate, 98–100, 99t, 100t
miscellaneous agents, 107–108
prostaglandin inhibition, 105
vasopressors, 100–101
physical measures for
head-up tilt at night, 95
lower body external pressure, 95, *96,* 97
mitral valve prolapse and, 42–44, 43t

neurogenic, 26–27, 27t, 28t
afferent lesions and, 27–28
central disorders and, 29
idiopathic parkinsonism, 29–30
miscellaneous causes, 30–31
Riley-Day syndrome (Familial dysautonomia), 30
disorders primarily affecting sympathetic chain and postganglionic nerves and
diabetes mellitus, 44–45
miscellaneous neuropathies, 45–47
efferent defects and, 31, 32t–33t, 34
idiopathic orthostatic hypotension, 34
multiple-system atrophy (Shy-Drager syndrome), 35–38
miscellaneous lesions in the spinal cord and, 44
orthostatic hypotension and mitral valve prolapse and, 42–44, 43t
orthostatic hypotension associated with excessive sympathetic discharge (sympathicotonic orthostatic hypotension), and 41–42
pathology and pathogenesis of multiple-system atrophy and idiopathic orthostatic hypotension and, 38–39, *40,* 41
pathophysiologic and pharmacologic investigations of, 55–57, *56*
antidiuretic hormone (arginine vasopressin) and, 61–62
enzyme measurements and, 62
plasma catecholamine studies and, 57, 58t, 59
pressor agent infusions and, 59–61, 60t, 62–63
spinal cord lesions and, 44
sympathetic chain and postganglionic nerve disorders and
diabetes mellitus, 44–45
miscellaneous neuropathies, 45–47

PANHYPOPITUITARISM, orthostatic hypotension and, 21
Parkinsonism, idiopathic, neurogenic orthostatic hypotension and, 29–30
Pathogenesis and pathology of multiple-system atrophy, 38–39, *40,* 41
Pathology and pathogenesis of multiple-system atrophy, 38–39, *40,* 41

Pathophysiologic and pharmacologic investigations of neurogenic orthostatic hypotension, 55–57, *56*
  antidiuretic hormone (arginine vasopressin) and, 61–62
  enzyme measurements and, 62
  plasma catecholamine studies and, 57, 58t, 59
  postsynaptic adrenergic receptors and, 61
  pressor agent infusions and, 59–61, 60t, 62–63
Patient history, clinical diagnosis of orthostatic hypotension and, 72–74, 73t
Perfusion, inadequate arterial, clinical diagnosis of orthostatic hypotension and symptoms of, 69–70
Peripheral vasculature defects, orthostatic hypotension and
  congenital defect in norepinephrine release, 48
  hyperbradykininism and, 47–48
Pharmacologic agents, orthostatic hypotension due to, 19–20
Pharmacologic and pathophysiologic investigations of neurogenic orthostatic hypotension
  antidiuretic hormone (arginine vasopressin) and, 61–62
  plasma catecholamine studies and, 57, 58t, 59
  postsynaptic adrenergic receptors and, 61
  pressor agent infusions and, 59–61, 60t, 62–63
Pharmacologic measures, management of orthostatic hypotension and, 97–98, 98t
  adrenergic blockers, 105–107
  ergot derivatives, 102, 103t, 104t
  fludrocortisone acetate, 98–100, 99t, 100t
  miscellaneous agents, 107–108
  prostaglandin inhibition, 105
  vasopressors, 100–101
Phenylephrine, management of orthostatic hypotension and, 100–101
Phenylephrine hydrochloride injection, clinical diagnosis of orthostatic hypotension and, 83
Physical measures for management of orthostatic hypotension
  head-up tilt at night, 95
  lower body external pressure, 95, *96*, 97

Physical examination, clinical diagnosis of orthostatic hypotension and, 73t, 74–76
Physical exertion, orthostatic hypotension and, 15
Pindolol, management of orthostatic hypotension and, 106–107
Plasma catecholamine studies, neurogenic orthostatic hypotension and, 57, 58t, 59
Postganglionic nerve and sympathetic chain disorders, orthostatic hypotension and
  diabetes mellitus, 44–45
  miscellaneous neuropathies, 45–47
Postsynaptic adrenergic receptors, neurogenic orthostatic hypotension and, 61
Postural adjustment, inadequate, orthostatic hypotension and
  aging and, 16–17
  asthenic habitus with poorly developed musculature and, 15
  bed rest and/or space flight and, 15–16
  miscellaneous causes and, 17–18
    anorexia nervosa, 17
    fever, 18
    gastrectomy, 17
    marijuana use, 18
    pregnancy, 17
  physical exertion and, 15
Pregnancy, orthostatic hypotension during, 17
Prenalterol, management of orthostatic hypotension and, 101
Pressor agent infusions, neurogenic orthostatic hypotension and, 59–61, 60t, 62–63
Pressure, lower body external, management of orthostatic hypotension and, 95, *96*, 97
Prolapse, mitral valve
  case study of sympathicotonic orthostatic hypotension and, 115–116
  orthostatic hypotension and, 42–44, 43t
Propranolol, management of orthostatic hypotension and, 105–106
Prostaglandin inhibition, management of orthostatic hypotension and, 105
Prosthesis, sympathetic neural, management of orthostatic hypotension and, 108–109

RECEPTORS, postsynaptic adrenergic, neurogenic orthostatic hypotension and, 61

Reflex arteriolar constriction, maintenance of normal blood pressure upon standing and, 2–6, *4, 5*
Reflex venous constriction, maintenance of normal blood pressure upon standing and, 6
Renin-angiotensin-aldosterone system, maintenance of normal blood pressure upon standing and, 8
Respiratory and muscle changes, maintenance of normal blood pressure upon standing and, 10
Riley-Day syndrome, neurogenic orthostatic hypotension and, 30

Shy-Drager syndrome. *See also* Multiple-system atrophy
  neurogenic orthostatic hypotension and, 35–38
Space flight, orthostatic hypotension and, 15–16
Spinal cord lesions, orthostatic hypotension and, 44
Standing
  heart rate response to, clinical diagnosis of orthostatic hypotension and, 81–82
  maintenance of normal blood pressure and, 1–2, 2t, *3*
    cerebral blood flow and, 9–10
    hormonal responses and, 8
    increase in heart rate and, *3,* 6–8, 7
    reflex arteriolar constriction and, 2–6, *4, 5*
    reflex venous constriction and, 6
    respiratory and muscle changes and, 10
  vasopressin response to, clinical diagnosis of orthostatic hypotension and, 83
Sweat tests, clinical diagnosis of orthostatic hypotension and, 84–85
Sympathetic chain and postganglionic nerve disorders, orthostatic hypotension and
  diabetes mellitus, 44–45
  miscellaneous neuropathies, 45–47
Sympathetic discharge, excessive, orthostatic hypotension and, 41–42
Sympathetic neural prosthesis, management of orthostatic hypotension and, 108–109
Sympathicotonic orthostatic

hypotension, case study of mitral valve prolapse and, 115–116
Syndrome
  Riley-Day, neurogenic orthostatic hypotension and, 30
  Shy-Drager, neurogenic orthostatic hypotension and, 35–38

TACHYPACING, atrial, management of orthostatic hypotension and, 107–108
Tests
  afferent function, clinical diagnosis of orthostatic hypotension and
    amyl nitrate inhalation, 82
    heart rate response to standing, 81–82
    phenylephrine hydrochloride injection, 83
    vasopressin response to standing, 83
  autonomic function, clinical diagnosis of orthostatic hypotension and, 78, 79t
    modified noninvasive Valsalva maneuver, 81
    Valsalva maneuver, 78, *80,* 80–81
  central function, clinical diagnosis of orthostatic hypotension and, 83–84
  efferent function, clinical diagnosis of orthostatic hypotension and
    invasive
      norepinephrine infusion, 86–87
      tyramine infusion, 86
    noninvasive
      arithmetic under stress, 84
      cold pressor test, 84
      epinephrine instillation into the eye, 85
      plasma norepinephrine levels, 85–86
      sweat tests, 84–85
Tyramine
  infusion of
    clinical diagnosis of orthostatic hypotension and, 86
    orthostatic hypotension and, 59–60, 60t
  management of orthostatic hypotension and, 101

VALSALVA maneuver, clinical diagnosis of orthostatic hypotension and, 78, *80,* 80–81
  modified noninvasive, 81
Vanillylmandelic acid, maintenance of normal blood pressure upon standing and, 8
Vasculature, peripheral, defects in, orthostatic hypotension and

Vasculature, peripheral, defects in, orthostatic hypotension and—*continued*
congenital defect in norepinephrine release, 48
hyperbradykininism and, 47–48
Vasopressin, arginine
maintenance of normal blood pressure upon standing and, 8
neurogenic orthostatic hypotension and, 61–62
Vasopressors, management of orthostatic hypotension and, 100–101
Venous constriction, reflex, maintenance of normal blood pressure upon standing and, 6
VMA. *See* Vanillylmandelic acid